How to Help Non-Speaking Children in the Early Years

In every setting, there are children who struggle to communicate. When they're not talking, or only using a handful of words, it can be hard to know how to help. In this book, you'll be encouraged to spot early moments of communication and respond with clarity. You'll find an invitation to stop doing and start noticing, to try new things, and collaborate with the team around you.

The book presents key concepts in bite-sized chunks, with a wealth of real-life examples from speech therapy sessions and early years settings. It explores practical strategies to help children develop their foundational speech, language and communication skills, and includes fresh ideas to:

- Build honest and supportive conversations with parents about communication needs
- Value empathy and imagination as we tune in to each child's world
- Take a pro-neurodiversity lens to inform your practice
- Measure progress and support professional development

Communication is core to our sense of wellbeing, personal agency and belonging. With a focus on fostering joyful moments of connection, this book offers a fresh perspective and a dose of encouragement for all early years practitioners, speech and language therapists, SENCOs, and key people looking to develop the communication skills of children in their care.

If you care for a young child who isn't speaking, or is using just a handful of words, this book will give you an accessible starting guide to connect and communicate together with joy.

Bryony Rust, aka SaLT by the Sea, is a speech and language therapist sharing her own experiences of what works with young children, learned through years of providing therapy, training practitioners, and collaborating with caregivers. Bryony is also a keynote speaker and clinical supervisor, helping others navigate the surprise delights and challenges of helping young children learn to talk. To find out more, visit saltbythesea.com

"Bryony's book is an absolute must-read for any parent, teacher, professional, educator or caregiver looking to better connect and communicate with children, especially non-verbal or neurodivergent kids. This wonderfully practical and accessible guide is filled with creative strategies to try, garnered from Bryony's own practice and research. Her friendly, understanding and non-judgemental tone throughout the book helps to put you at your ease as you embark on the journey of tuning into your child's world, whether you have a verbal child, a late talker, or a child with additional needs. Bryony invites us to reflect on what makes our best interactions and relationships so special and reminds us that these sacred spaces of connection should be the core aim for speech therapy, not chasing arbitrary targets. You'll be liberated to slow down, let the child take the lead, and embrace any and all forms of communication that arise naturally through play. This book will help you to reflect on your interactions and expand your understanding of what it means to communicate meaningfully with children. I highly recommend this brilliant book - it's an investment in deepening your bond with your child in beautifully life-changing ways."

– **Kathy Brodie**, Early Years Consultant and Founder of Early Years TV

"A witty, compassionate and honest guide to nurturing communication. This book is for all non-speaking children and any person who supports them. Bryony's strength based view of ability shines through whilst offering quality exercises and reflections to try out in practice."

– **Lyra Wright**, Early Childhood Teacher

"This is a glorious, gentle book that will be supportive, accepting and inspiring to parents/carers and professionals. A book that truly encourages us to place the child at the centre of care but also that and acknowledges the challenging, but oh so valuable, role of parents and carers."

– **Suzanne Churcher**, Speech and Language Therapist and Lecturer, University of Sheffield

"Bryony writes from a personal and experienced perspective as a Speech and Language Therapist with joy, passion and insight. Her advice is approachable and compassionate."
— **Louise Coigley**, Speech and Language Therapist, Lis'n Tell: Live Inclusive Storytelling

"Bryony lays out a perspective shift for how to follow a child's lead and increase connection and joy to facilitate communication. From child-led therapy, to observing the child, to being a communication partner that follows (rather than leads), this book lays out the 'how to' of interaction that is fun, playful and facilitates language and connection for the children we work with."
— **Sarah Lockhart**, M.S. CCC-SLP, SLP Happy Hour

"What a joy to read. I urge anyone of whatever level of experience, to read this book. From initial Speech and Language Therapy training to CPD, it will encourage your reflective practice and make you an even better you. Bryony's book helps to peel back the layers to find (or rediscover) the important core when supporting non-speaking children. It emphasises the importance of the child, waiting for them to lead and being ok with silence. Through recognisable examples, Bryony shows us how we can word things differently, refocussing on small things that can make a big difference, providing many practical 'take homes' throughout. This book reminds us to 'trust in the value of what the child shows you'; I am grateful for the reminder and for this gift of a book.
— **Sarah Parsons**, Speech and Language Therapist, Redriff Primary City of London Academy

*"This book really made me reflect on my own practice with families and children (not just non-speaking ones). Bryony has crafted something that is accessible and full of optimism, while being frank about the challenges. Addressing so many of the questions and challenges that families and practitioners ask about, in a non-judgemental, practical, kind way, this is useful reading for parents, family members, practitioners

and SLTs alike. I really loved the suggestions on goal setting, strength-based descriptions of communication and the practical strategies. I'm never going to be able to listen to Daft Punk again without thinking of the washing machine song!"

– **Rachel Tuckely**, Specialist Speech and Language Therapist, Sound Talk Speech and Language Therapy Ltd

"Bryony so beautifully weaves her professional insights and personal anecdotes to share the importance of a child led and strengths based focus when supporting communication, play and connection. This book was full of hope, joy and celebration of non-speaking children. Honouring and appreciating their ideas, attempts to communicate, and meeting them where they are at in order to support their speech and language, play, and ongoing development. I finished the book feeling like it is a permission slip to slow down, get attentive and really listen to what children are telling us."

– **Carly Budd**, Occupational Therapist and Founder of Developmental Play Academy

"A refreshingly empathic personal perspective, focusing on a child led approach to communicating with non-speaking children."

– **Lou. E,** Approved Foster Carer for 10+ Years

"A breath of fresh air. Focussing on the relationship first, Bryony sets out thoughts, frameworks and strategies that are child-led, celebratory and meaningful – focussing on connection, collaboration and most importantly, fun! Using examples and analogies throughout, she explores a range of considerations and urges us to think about things differently - including the importance of co-regulation, shifting our language to be more strengths based, and embracing awkward silences! As she rightly states, communication is "about so much more than words."

– **Frances Johnstone**, Founder and Director of Therapy Links UK CIC, Principal Speech and Language Therapist

"This is a beautifully written, warm hug of a book, which gently informs and facilitates reflection on how to help non-speaking children with a kind, difference-affirming approach. The narrative "it's ok to try stuff and don't worry if it goes wrong sometimes" will appeal to parents and practitioners alike. The honest and touching stories of challenges Bryony has faced in her own life, interwoven into the text, make the book entirely relatable. I found myself thinking "yes – exactly that" at many points. I wish I'd had this book earlier in my career and will absolutely recommend it to parents, SLT students and supervisees."

– **Jan Baerselman**, Director, Talking Outcomes Speech & Language Consultancy

"This wonderful little book is a fabulous storied account of the ethos of supporting and scaffolding shared moments of connection with people. It is beautifully written, and absorbed quickly and easily. I will recommend it to every speech and language therapy student that I meet. The principles and strategies apply, not just to children in the early years, but to anyone who finds communication difficult at any time in their lives."

– **Jo Sandiford**, Senior Lecturer and Speech and Language Therapist, Leeds

How to Help Non-Speaking Children in the Early Years

Supporting Communication through Joy and Connection

Bryony Rust

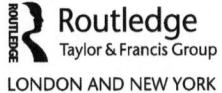

LONDON AND NEW YORK

Designed cover image: Victoria Escandell

First published 2025
by Routledge
4 Park Square, Milton Park, Abingdon, Oxon OX14 4RN

and by Routledge
605 Third Avenue, New York, NY 10158

Routledge is an imprint of the Taylor & Francis Group, an informa business

© 2025 Bryony Rust

Illustrations by Victoria Escandell

The right of Bryony Rust to be identified as author of this work has been asserted in accordance with sections 77 and 78 of the Copyright, Designs and Patents Act 1988.

All rights reserved. No part of this book may be reprinted or reproduced or utilised in any form or by any electronic, mechanical, or other means, now known or hereafter invented, including photocopying and recording, or in any information storage or retrieval system, without permission in writing from the publishers.

Trademark notice: Product or corporate names may be trademarks or registered trademarks, and are used only for identification and explanation without intent to infringe.

British Library Cataloguing-in-Publication Data
A catalogue record for this book is available from the British Library

ISBN: 9781032295176 (hbk)
ISBN: 9781032295190 (pbk)
ISBN: 9781003301967 (ebk)

DOI: 10.4324/9781003301967

Typeset in Optima LT Std
by Deanta Global Publishing Services, Chennai, India

Contents

1	**What this guide is and how it can help you**	**1**
	What we're aiming for	1
	Stop doing, start noticing	2
	What to expect from this book	4
2	**Expand your definition of communication**	**6**
	Speech, language, and communication	6
	Talking isn't everything	8
	Always respond	12
	Understand why we bother	14
	Look out for opportunities	15
	Understand what's going on behind the scenes	17
	Why do some kids find talking so hard?	19
3	**Build relationships**	**22**
	Include everyone from the beginning	22
	Aim for a flat hierarchy	24
	Practise active listening	28
	Avoid fix-it mode	30

CONTENTS

	Stay out of judgement	32
	Realise our shared humanity	34
	'Celebrate with me'	35
4	**Start from strength**	**37**
	Tell a story of hope	37
	Describe what the child can do	40
	Remember they're in the room	43
	Shift your language from disorder to difference	43
	Respect at all times	44
	Consider needs, not problems	45
	Trust in capacity	46
5	**Let the child lead**	**49**
	Tune in to the child's point of interest	49
	Give it space	52
	Look for the invitations	54
	Directing vs. responding	54
	Give attention to get attention	57
	Solutions for when it's hard	58
6	**Choose your focus**	**63**
	Decide what's important	63
	A note on mindfulness	65
	Understand where the child's at	70
	Write goals for the adults, not the child	72
	Write SCRUFFY goals	74

7	**A strategies list**	**77**
	Allow yourself to do less	78
	Embrace the awkward silence	78
	Reflect the child	80
	Pay attention to the details	82
	Play with words	83
	Use big gestures	86
	Make your phrases sing	87
	Use sound effects	89
	Give, don't quiz	89
	Make it easy	90
	Eye contact: A word of caution	91
8	**Keep going**	**93**
	Imagine something different	93
	We're in the business of relationships	95
	The simple version	96
	Share with others	97
	Choose one thing	97
	Stick with it	98
	Embrace everything	99
	It's all in the noticing	101
	Useful links	*103*
	Acknowledgements	*104*
	Index	*105*

What this guide is and how it can help you

What we're aiming for

It seems to me a wonder that we're able to share so many rich, complex ideas together. How incredible that we should have thoughts in our heads and find so many ways to get them out into the world and hear others respond. With all that's involved in communicating, so many intricate steps, it's a marvel that we manage it at all. It's useful and it's downright joyful to connect with someone and find shared sentiment. No wonder we want that for our children too. We experience the everyday magic and necessity of communicating with others. We know how essential communication is for each child. We see the everyday impact when they struggle.

At a basic level, it's important that our kids can understand what we're telling them, so they can make sense of the world and their daily routines. It's important that they can tell us what they need, tell us when they're scared, hungry, hurt. But it's also much more than that. Communication is core to our sense of wellbeing, personal agency, and belonging. We've all experienced the wounded feeling when our communication isn't 'right'.

I was an exuberant kid; always moving, singing and hollering. I loved pastel purples and those candy necklaces. When I was four, I moved with my family across the Atlantic to Scotland. We left hot and sunny California and landed in a very different climate. I remember sitting on the carpet of my new classroom and getting things wrong. I said 'sandwiches' differently at registration, the other kids sniggered. I quickly learned that my voice was too loud and my words sounded wrong, so I retreated into a defensive shell of not-quite-fitting-in.

My experience of being the outsider was trifling in comparison to so many, but it's the personal experience that we have to draw on. Through this book, I'll encourage you to do the same. Empathy is key to how we connect and start to tune in to each child's world.

Do our non-speaking children also experience a sense of not-quite-rightness? And if so, can we prioritise time to embrace and celebrate them without an undercurrent of deficit? This book is an invitation to explore just that: what to do when a child isn't matching the communication development of their peers. How to enable joyful moments of connection together and support communication development.

Stop doing, start noticing

When I first trained as a speech and language therapist back in the noughties, I felt a great deal of pressure to have all the answers, to be busy fixing. When families brought their little one to a clinic appointment, I kicked into gear, pulling out all the whizz-bang-flash toys, trying all the prompts and enticements to get each child to talk.

I tried to make the most of a short appointment at the end of a very long waiting list, to be efficient and speedy right at a point when that family most needed patience and time. Some of my sessions ended in tug-of-war battles, full meltdowns, or silent standoffs. If it's happened to you, you can bet it's happened to me.

Over the years, my approach has shifted to one of greater patience and genuine curiosity about what each child wants to engage in. Learning from a variety of therapeutic approaches and teachers, I started exploring what would happen if I didn't *drive* the interaction. It wasn't always an easy shift. The challenge to pause and leave more space for the child to lead was genuinely scary. If I wasn't directing and entertaining, then where was my value? How could this child learn if I wasn't leading? How were we going to get anything 'done'?! Discomfort aside, as I became less directive and gave each child more time to think and take the lead, I noticed how they filled the space that I gave them, how they used it to think more deeply and reach out to me to share their ideas. The less I directed, the more I was able to follow their lead. I found myself in a better position to notice and support where the child was at.

We're going to look at how we can genuinely follow a child's lead and why we should bother in the first place. Not only because increased engagement = stronger learning. But because, over time, we see the natural process of learning unfold. We see how our active attention and intentional responses, are sufficient to support their development, without us having to direct or plan a 'learning activity'.

I know I'm not alone in feeling the pressure to be busy doing, to direct a child's actions and attention. This feeling often intensifies when a child doesn't show us the familiar steps of early communication: gesturing, copying words and sounds, paying attention to what we show them. We think we're somehow not doing enough to 'make it work'. So we get even busier, or we abandon with the very understandable reasoning that the child just prefers to spend time alone.

In this book, I want to give you permission to do less. Less directing, less planning, less testing. I want you to see the enormous value in those moments when you can sit alongside a child and pay attention to the tiny details of what they're doing. That's how we give kids the space and permission to reach out to us and show us how they see the world.

And why should that matter? Beyond all our busy plans and activities, we all need a sense of belonging. Finding a way to communicate what feels important to you is a central aspect of wellbeing. We want each child to learn that their ideas matter, that it's worth the effort to share them with us.

Ultimately, my hope for these growing humans is that they have a sense of freedom to be themselves, speak up, and be in relation with others in a way that is mutually kind and creative. This is how we find community and our place in the world.

Communication skills help us face challenges collaboratively and find solutions that help us thrive. It is possible to approach our interactions with young children in the same way we would a human at any age: with respectful attention, appreciation, and understanding. After all, so many of the communication skills we help our children develop are things we refine over a lifetime: sharing space, attending to others, asking for help, receiving suggestions, adapting, and collaborating. We can all benefit from a focus on mutual understanding, genuine appreciation, and non-judgemental curiosity.

What to expect from this book

I'm a cisgender, able-bodied white woman, who is not a parent. All of this impacts my experience and perspectives. I don't consider myself an expert. This book is not a textbook or a thesis. It's my personal perspective, gained not just from my training as a speech and language therapist, but also the countless hours I've spent with young kids and their caregivers, and the supportive conversations I've had along the way.

The ideas shared in this book are formed from my own professional development and this is a collection of what I know so far. I'm always learning and adjusting, and I hope that will forever be the case. Reflective practice and collaborative working is a priority in speech therapy for a reason. There will never be 'one right way' to nurture children's development and we need to keep sharing our perspectives and learn from each other.

I hope that this book can be a conversation with you as the reader. Because your experiences and skills may differ from mine, and that makes them all the more valuable. We all have ideas to contribute to our work helping kids communicate.

There are reflective questions scattered throughout the book. Feel free to write in the margins, or pause and take time to jot down your thoughts. However you choose to chew on this book, I encourage you to write something down. That is a really powerful part of how we take meaningful action from what we read.

Together, we'll look at the details of what developing communication skills look like for young children. When we know what we're looking for we're better placed to notice and respond in a way that's helpful. We'll look at the kind of responses we can practise that support a child's growth. We'll look at what's really going on between the two of you in those moments of 'not doing very much'.

We're focusing here on laying a foundation for strong attunement between the child and the adult. These early principles for shared attention, engagement, and enjoyment, support a child's development, regardless of whether the primary need is one around articulating sounds, using words, or communicating with others. That said, this book has a focus on the kids I meet who are not talking, or using only a handful of spoken words.

I hope the ideas here give you a sense of possibility and joy in your interactions with young children. Our kids learn better when we're having fun together and we feel better about our work when we're enjoying it. Whether the work of supporting a non-speaking child is yours as a professional, a caregiver, or a supportive community member, it is important and valuable.

I hope to give you permission to get playful together and find the things that spark joy for you both, knowing that this is how we help children flourish. You won't hear mention of rewards or stickers. Communication shouldn't need a bribe. Sharing messages and interacting with others can be intrinsically rewarding, not something that we need to coax out of a child, but instead something that we can be available for and ready to facilitate.

We can be playful, curious, and open communication partners. We can be imaginative as we wonder about the world from a child's perspective. We can be active listeners and willing teammates, sharing our own perspectives and learning alongside all the other adults in a child's life. No one has all the answers. This whole messy business of communication is about working things out together.

This is why I approach my interactions with children with a sense of open enquiry. What will we discover today? I won't be giving you a prescribed protocol or a step-by-step list of instructions. Instead, I'm giving you an open invitation to explore and experiment. Try out the ideas shared in this book, chat with others about what you notice and build on this together. Kids need someone who can notice, reflect, and adapt to the beautiful variety of communication styles out there. I think you're just that person.

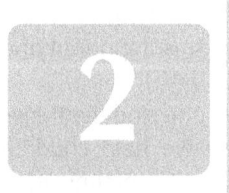

Expand your definition of communication

Speech, language, and communication

> Can you think of a time when you had a really good conversation with someone? Jot down or close your eyes and imagine the details of that experience. What was it about this interaction that felt good to you? How did it make you feel?

Perhaps you felt listened to, or perhaps you felt like you were having fun together. Maybe it felt unhurried, like you had time to really get into a deep chat together.

When we reflect on our own experiences and dig into the feelings behind it, we can find inspiration for how we want our kids to feel within their interactions with us.

We don't think much about communication until it goes wrong. Those moments of misunderstanding can be uncomfortable and often inevitable. How could we possibly get it right all the time when there's so many intricate parts at play? When we communicate, we have to pay attention to someone else, listen carefully to what they're saying and how they're saying it, notice our own internal reactions, think about how to respond and what to say next. This remains true whether you're two or 92, although the details may look different.

So, what about those details? In the world of speech and language therapy, there are important distinctions in how we define *speech*, *language*, and *communication*.

EXPAND YOUR DEFINITION OF COMMUNICATION

> Do you know the difference between speech, language and communication? Jot down your ideas and then reflect on how they match up with these descriptions.

Speech is about the sounds that we make with our mouths to produce words. If a child has speech difficulties, they may be struggling to produce a range of sounds, which impacts on how clearly they speak.

Language is about words and sentences. It includes details around vocabulary, sentence construction, and comprehension. If a child has language difficulties, they might struggle to learn new words, or they might find it hard to put those words into sentences. Language difficulties also impact a child's ability to understand what you're saying to them.

Communication is the big picture. It includes the many additional skills involved in understanding one another: thinking about the other person, noticing and using body language, different tones of voice, facial expressions, and more. Communication is about learning how to be around other people and share ideas together. We can communicate a lot of information without using words.

This whole business of communicating with someone involves a complex sequence of skills (as summarised in Figure 2.1).

To express ourselves, we have to generate thoughts, think about how to form these into words and phrases, produce the individual speech sounds to articulate these words and phrases. We also have to think about the listener: judge whether they're paying attention to us, consider how they might receive our message.

And communication isn't just about expressing ourselves. We also need to be able to receive the other person's message. We need to process the sounds we hear, understand the words they form, and hold all that information in our working memory long enough to understand the message formed from all those sounds and words.

It can be useful to separate the individual skills ('attention, comprehension, expression … vocabulary, social thinking, articulation …') and lay them out as a linear process, so we can examine them, and chart progress. That approach informs our direction and focus, but it's not the whole picture. It's a complex, interlinked and nonlinear process. Communication is far more broad and beautiful than we could ever capture in boxes.

HOW TO HELP NON-SPEAKING CHILDREN IN THE EARLY YEARS

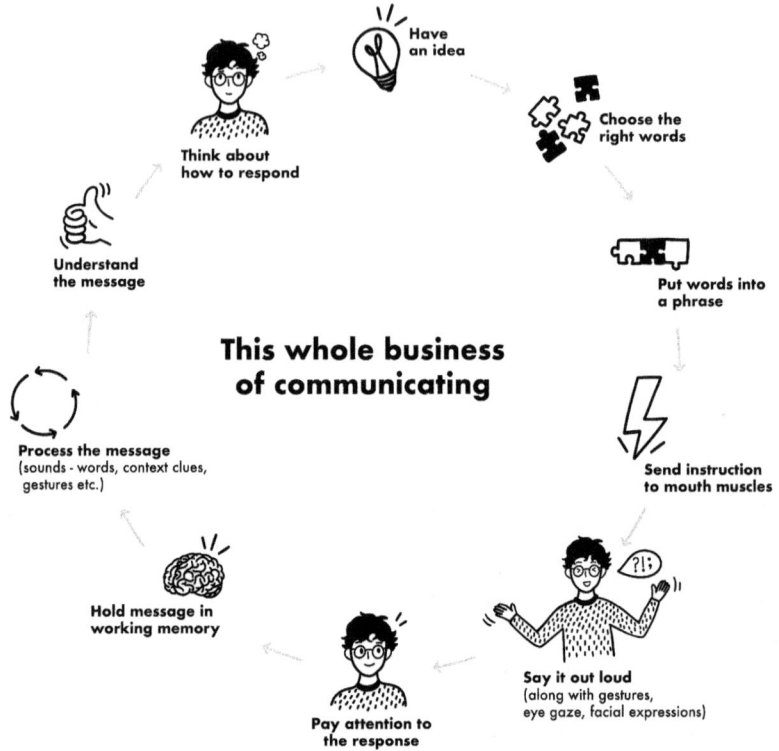

Figure 2.1 An abbreviated illustration of the many interlinking skills involved in communicating with others

Communication is a messy, dynamic thing between people. It's not possible to simply follow a checklist and know we've completed the steps to effective communication. If it were, we wouldn't experience all those cringey moments when it goes awry. Communication is play and experimentation, trial and error.

Talking isn't everything

The simplified sequence above focuses on the talking. That's how we convey a lot of our thoughts and feelings, but it's not everything. We can communicate a lot with a frown or a shout, a point or a wiggle. When we hail a bus or ask for two more at the bar, when we show scepticism about someone's idea or celebrate their success – our bodies are involved in all of those communications, in a rich variety of ways.

Additional ways in which a child might communicate:

- Gesture
- Voice
- Facial expression
- Body proximity (coming in close, or backing away)
- Eye gaze
- Body movements
- Laughter!

When you consider all this natural, unspoken communication, alongside our everyday use of pictures and symbols (following road signs, finding the loo, using our phones) it's clear we are all multimodal communicators. Children

Whole body communication

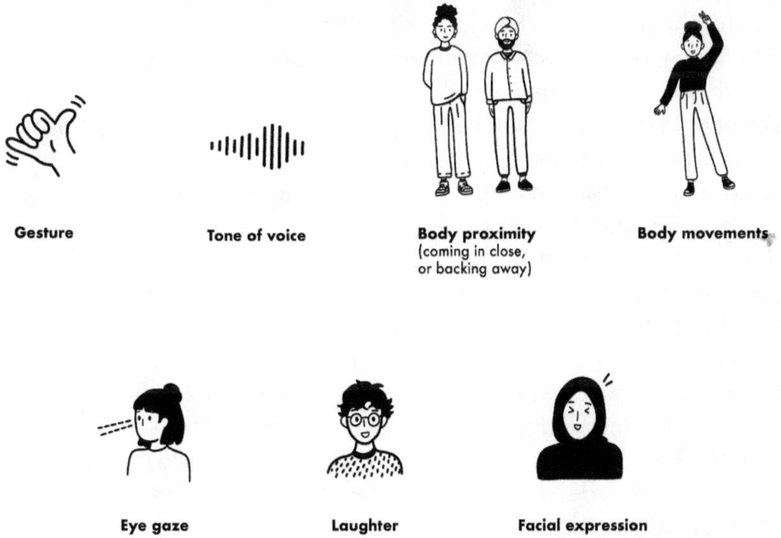

Gesture · Tone of voice · Body proximity (coming in close, or backing away) · Body movements

Eye gaze · Laughter · Facial expression

Figure 2.2 Some of the common ways we communicate with our bodies

learn to communicate multimodally, too. That becomes all the more important, and worth paying attention to, when a child isn't using much spoken language.

When families come to speech and language therapy, they typically share a primary goal. They will say they want to hear more words. Of course! The world opens up when we can talk with others, and we want that for our kids.

But talking isn't always first on the agenda. There are many other elements to consider, that are just as important to how we communicate with each other. Some kids need time to establish the foundations: sharing space, noticing and attending to one another, exploring tone of voice. Learning how a face can change shape, and be mirrored in the face of someone else. Exploring the way our hands move, how we can combine this with sounds and words. These are just a few of the things we can explore when we interact. For some, that takes time and energy to absorb.

Add to that the processing demands of any environment: the background sounds, the movement of people around, the sights and smells. All of that takes energy too, and not everyone processes sensory information in the same way. Sometimes when a child I meet is particularly averse to something, or unusually interested in something, I start by imagining that they may be perceiving this whole situation differently. Their sensory profile (sight, touch, sound, taste, movement, and more) may not match mine at all.

When F and his parents came to visit me in my clinic, he was really interested in the beep in the hallway. I don't know for how long it had been beeping, prior to F's first visit, because I had never noticed it, until his own glance and vocalisations drew my attention to it. After they left that first session, I was out there in the hallway, leaning down and then stretching up on my tip toes, trying to locate that mysterious beep. It had just the right intermittency to feel like your brain might be inventing it, and certainly just the right volume to make it hard to find.

Turns out, it was a smoke alarm that needed a new battery. And over the first few weeks that F visited me, he would notice the beep in the hallway and I would acknowledge it. He would glance towards the sound, then copy the beep. Then I would make a beep sound, too. He would look towards me when I made the sound. He started to respond to my 'beep' with an expression that read 'You hear it too!' Then he started saying 'beep' after me. Over time, we had built a little exchange, like batting a ball back and forth.

We didn't focus on the talking. We focused on what interested him, meeting him where he was at. I focused on responding through sound, gesture and looks. By doing that, I extended a bridge to give him a way to 'talk' about the thing he found interesting. It felt kind of minimal. It also made the space pretty quiet. And that meant that the thing of interest, this hidden little beep in the hallway, could be heard. And F had things to say about it.

Eventually, the battery was changed and our 'in joke' or shared exchange ended. But, by then, we'd developed several other shared exchanges, and more nuanced intentional ways of moving and vocalising to communicate.

His parents took video clips on their phone, and I caught short clips on a camcorder. This video record is one of the most powerful ways that his parents and I were able to talk about and support his progress over time. It's hard to translate these developments in to words, because they involve so few of them!

Little F is speaking now, and he's not so little. I almost hesitate to share his longer term progress towards speaking, because it draws our thoughts away from the importance of valuing the unspoken and taking time to establish the other parts of communication.

There's a practice in allowing for the fact that the interactions, the 'chat' that you're having with a child is not 'word-heavy'. It has an element of mindfulness about it: being ok with the quiet subtleties of the moment. But, more on that in Chapter 6.

We need the time and space to appreciate shared engagement, sustained focus, and shifting attention. Together, we need to discover the things that we can *both* attend to, share thoughts on, through our actions and vocalisations, our faces and hands. Expanding our awareness of all that's involved in communication helps us notice and value the non-spoken as much as the spoken. The very act of doing this allows these foundation skills to flourish.

When I highlight the value of the unspoken, I'm not suggesting that words are irrelevant. We can still be intentional about the words we model to children. But, if that's our primary focus, we're at risk of missing other important (and fun!) parts of how we interact with one another.

If we focus only on words, we miss other moments we could respond to, the ways that a child is already reaching out and conveying something. We miss the opportunity to connect with what they are doing, without striving for something different. Allowing for what is, rather than wanting something different, feels comfier in the body. That comfort conveys to the child: 'You're fine as you are, right here, and I'm here, and you don't have to *be* anything different. We're learning together.'

We need to be able to imagine a child's perspective, imagine what they may like to say about the situation and warmly respond to the varied ways in which they might be attempting to do so.

Always respond

You may come across the suggestion to do nothing until a child 'uses her words'. There's a fear that if you accept and respond to the non-spoken ways a child is communicating, then you could make them 'lazy' and they simply won't bother talking. Thing is, if talking is possible for a child then they will do it readily; it's by far the easiest option. Communicating an idea non-verbally often requires more effort, or can feel frustrating.

Withholding your response to a child, especially when you know the message they're trying to convey, interrupts the natural flow of the interaction. How strange that we should pretend we didn't understand a message, when really we did. How strange that we should have such specific and limiting views of what is 'correct' in each situation. I want communication to feel easy and successful, even for the children who struggle to speak. That's how we keep a child coming back for more. It's how we help them get brave enough to try harder things.

Just like you do, I want to help each child to learn words and start talking, but this doesn't come from making communication further out of reach or withholding your helpful response. It comes from responding enthusiastically to their efforts and finding the moments of fun and engagement together.

We may not hear a child speak, but we can see their ideas play out. We can pay attention to the details of their actions and tune in to their perspective. Reaching for a toy up high, diving in for a big hug, grabbing a hand to request some help, looking around to see if we're still there. These are all important moments of communication.

When you respond to a child's small and varied attempts at communication, you make it more likely that they'll keep trying. Far from encouraging them to be lazy, you're giving them encouragement and permission to keep going. 'I hear you … tell me more.'

EXPAND YOUR DEFINITION OF COMMUNICATION

A focus on responding to the child also puts us in the right headspace to be following the child's lead (more on that in Chapter 5). Responses are never the first act. The first act needs to come from the child, when they do something to show us what they're paying attention to. That might be something interesting or worrying, painful or outrageous. When we notice a child communicating this to us (in the varied ways they can) we start to naturally have more exchanges together. We start to see their actions as carrying a message that is worth responding to.

There's a whole bunch of ways we can respond that builds communication. We can respond both with spoken language and with all kinds of non-verbal action. It matters more that you respond, rather than how you respond.

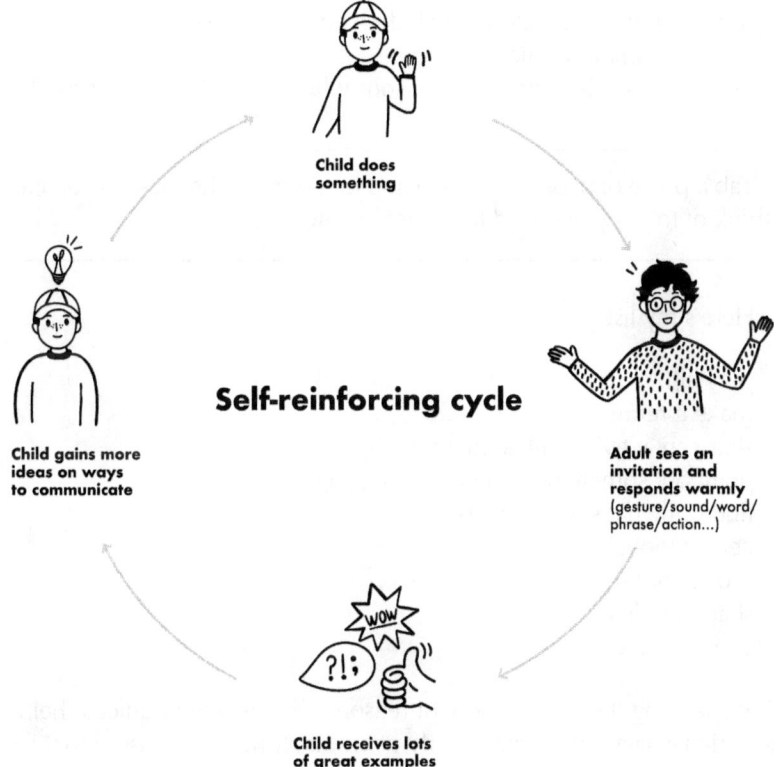

Figure 2.3 Our responses to children's communication attempts supports further communication attempts

Getting into the habit of responding to your child's tiny attempts is an important step in the process. The ways we respond to these efforts helps them learn whether they're on the right track. Over time, as your child becomes more sophisticated in their communication, so too will you become more confident in how you respond. We'll look more at the variety of ways you might respond in Chapter 7.

Understand why we bother

If this business of communication is so complex and difficult, why do we even bother? Communication can feel vulnerable, and there's no guarantee of getting it 'right'. But still we seek the connection and understanding that comes from communication.

There's all kinds of practical reasons why we need to communicate.

> Grab a piece of paper and a pen and jot down all the reasons you can think of for why we need to communicate.

Here's my list:

- get help
- make a request
- share an activity with someone
- point out something you find interesting
- find out what someone else thinks
- get someone's attention
- protest or reject
- share an idea
- express a feeling

Acknowledging the huge variety of reasons why we communicate helps us take a richer view of a child's early attempts. It helps us ensure that we're on the lookout for the variety of reasons they're communicating, rather than focusing only on their ability to make basic requests.

Functional needs, like asking for help or requesting an item, is only a thin sliver of the reasons why we communicate. Yes, our children need to be able to communicate their basic needs, but there isn't a hierarchy to this. If communication is about being with others, then learning to talk about what excites us is just as fundamental as asking for a snack or the toilet.

Communication should be inherently motivating. Being able to share in your delight at how that toy jumps or how the water splashes. To be able to share when you're feeling silly or to get Dad to make that cool sound again. Perhaps these are basic needs, too: not just to be fed and watered, but also to share and connect, find meaning together. These are all important aspects of early communication.

We want children to learn over time that figuring out how to share their ideas is worth the effort, because the experience of being heard is intrinsically rewarding.

While sounds and words (speech and language) is part of the picture, it's this business of interaction (communication) that is where so many of the riches are. Helping kids to explore and learn how their own actions can impact the world around them, influence what happens and how people respond to them.

I'm interested in helping children to explore how they interact with others, direct their messages effectively, find enjoyment in play with others. It's the ability to connect and relate that feels essential to being human. I want kids to learn that they can affect the world around them, communicate ideas to others, through sounds, words, gestures and more. Our job as supportive adults is to see these small moments for what they are (communication!) so that we can build on these early steps.

Once we have a sense of the potential reasons a child might be communicating with us, we're in a good position to pay attention to the details, tune into the underlying purpose and respond in a helpful way.

Look out for opportunities

If you sit down in a corner of any pre-school you will invariably have a bunch of curious kids approach to say hello, perhaps ask your name. These are the kids who get the greeting, maybe some brief conversation. If you don't know the child, you'll probably end up commenting on what they're wearing or doing. 'I like the stars on your trainers' or 'Wow, that hula hoop is really big!' They might launch into telling you that Dani is coming over for tea, you might respond with 'Oh that's exciting.' Or you might say something about what you're having for tea. Either way, without much effort, this child has heard from you models of all kinds of varied vocabulary, commentary, and enthusiastic response to what the child has initiated. When communication is easy, opportunities for practice happen all the time.

When kids aren't talking and appear really absorbed in their own play, they're far less likely to get these everyday communication opportunities with the people around them. They might get lots of questions and prompts. Because, let's be real, it's hard for us adults to be met with quiet. All of this means that the kids who struggle to interact with us get fewer spontaneous opportunities to practise.

We need to dial up our sensitivity to what constitutes communicative attempts, to be alert to the moments when a non-speaking child is reaching out to us, so that every child has opportunities for conversation. And I do mean conversation – widening our imagining of what conversation can be: this mutually enjoyable exchange between two people.

I can think of times when I've had genuine heartfelt exchanges with kids, just through 'heys and 'huhs', 'oohs' and 'ahs'. If your kid makes a sound or waves a hand, you can respond like they're taking their turn in the conversation. Oh! Huh. Oh really? Well, yeah. Woooazah!

When you respond as if their sounds are a meaningful part of a conversation between the two of you, you're helping them to explore and develop it further.

Laughing, looking, chuckling, frowning, shoulder shrugging. All of this is part of how we communicate together and have fun in the process.

Every kid needs the opportunity to practise the relational stuff with you: learning how to be around others, what feels good, what things we can share, and how. It has to be fun, not a drill. So I realise the irony of what I'm about to suggest.

Plan for some 'practice time'. Five minutes when you're going to sit down with the child and just hang. This isn't because communication happens only in a pre-set time, but it helps us give focus to practices that are new. It helps us build new habits, that later feed into our everyday behaviours.

If communication is hard for your child, then they may well need your focused attention in order to practice. It's not always easy to fit that into a busy day. So, while you look out for things to notice, respond to, and build on, consider that this may not be enough and you may need to *plan* for opportunities, even though you don't need to plan any activities. This may mean timetabling frequent points across the week when you can have some dedicated time together, somewhere without lots of distractions.

Understand what's going on behind the scenes

If we hear a child use a word only once or twice, we might imagine that they're just being stubborn when they don't try again. But if we view the situation from the child's perspective, and consider how challenging the art of talking may be for them, we can start to understand why that word they used once is hard to find again.

The month that I was drafting this chapter, I had my first surfing lesson. As an ocean-loving island-dweller, surfing was something I wanted to try. In doing so, I got another humbling experience of what it feels like to be a beginner, to find something tricky and slow-going.

In that first surf lesson, Eddie the instructor laid out all kinds of important skills I had to string together. Point by point, he layered on the things to remember: board position, paddle timing, pop-up sequence, body awareness, water safety, and overall attention. After a couple of hours, I was starting to work it out and attempting to peel myself up into a standing position, all knees and elbows like a collapsing clothes horse. I even managed it a few times – standing up on my floaty beginner's board, riding high in the shallow foamy water. But, by the end of that two-hour lesson, no matter how hard I tried, I couldn't stand up again. I promise you, I wasn't being lazy.

I was also having fun, which is an essential part of learning and motivation at any age. If I didn't enjoy lolling about in the waves, figuring out the steps and knowing it was ok for me to take time to learn, there's no way I would keep trying. When things are too hard, we tend to give up.

Even though standing up on the board was the obvious goal, I was busy figuring out lots of other essential elements: watching the waves, learning how they curl and shape over time, handling my board, getting comfortable with the depth and feel of being washed about in the water. If standing up on the board had been our only success criterion for that lesson, I would have left feeling like a failure, and maybe Eddie would have, too.

Perhaps that's what happens when kids struggle to communicate. We're focusing on the obvious goal of talking, when they're still busy working out all the steps under the surface. We're waiting for the words while they're still figuring out how to:

- regulate their energy and emotions in new situations
- share space with someone else
- notice and pay attention to those around them
- engage in a shared point of interest
- understand what's being communicated to them
- decide how to respond

If you'd seen me in the water on that first surfing lesson, you might have said I was being lazy, because I wasn't standing up on the board very much and a lot of the time I was basically lolling about in the water. You couldn't know how hard I was working under the surface.

I put it to you that no child is lazy when they don't speak. We're simply not seeing all the other things they're busy working on. The glimpses we see when they attempt a sound or gesture, are big for them, may be a Herculean effort for those kids who have speech, language, and communication difficulties. Additionally, the everyday environment can be extra tricky for some of our kids to process. They might be easily overwhelmed by newness or loudness, by light, smells, textures (i.e., sensory processing differences).

We're asking kids to keep working hard at a skill that for some can feel at the very edges of their capability. This is why it's so important to establish fun within our time together. That's the only way we can keep going at something that is hard.

As an adult, we rarely experience complete beginnerhood as often as our kids do. I'm glad when I get the chance, because it's harder than I remember. All the steps, all the considerations, all the coordination and attention on different things. And even when you manage a key step, the progress is never neat and steady.

Progress

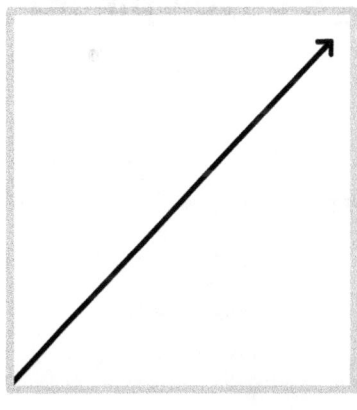
What we think progress looks like

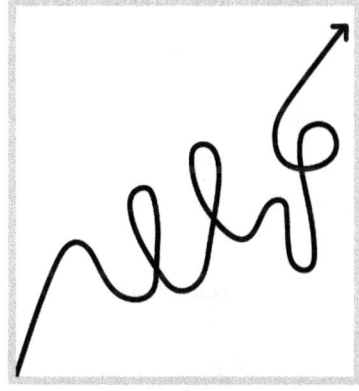
What progress actually looks like

Figure 2.4 What progress looks like

> REFLECT: What new skills have you recently tried to learn? What did you find hard? Were you surprised by how many hidden elements you had to work hard to apply? Might your own experiences as a beginner give you insight into how hard our kids are working?

It's easy to forget how hard it is to be a beginner. Learning any new skills involves consciously working through a lot of things that later become almost automatic. In some areas, we acquire skills easily, at other times we need extra help.

Why do some kids find talking so hard?

Spend any time with children and you'll see how they develop in different ways and at different paces. Sometimes the contrast in development can seem dramatic. 'I know I shouldn't compare but ...' is a phrase I often hear.

Factors that can impact speech and language development

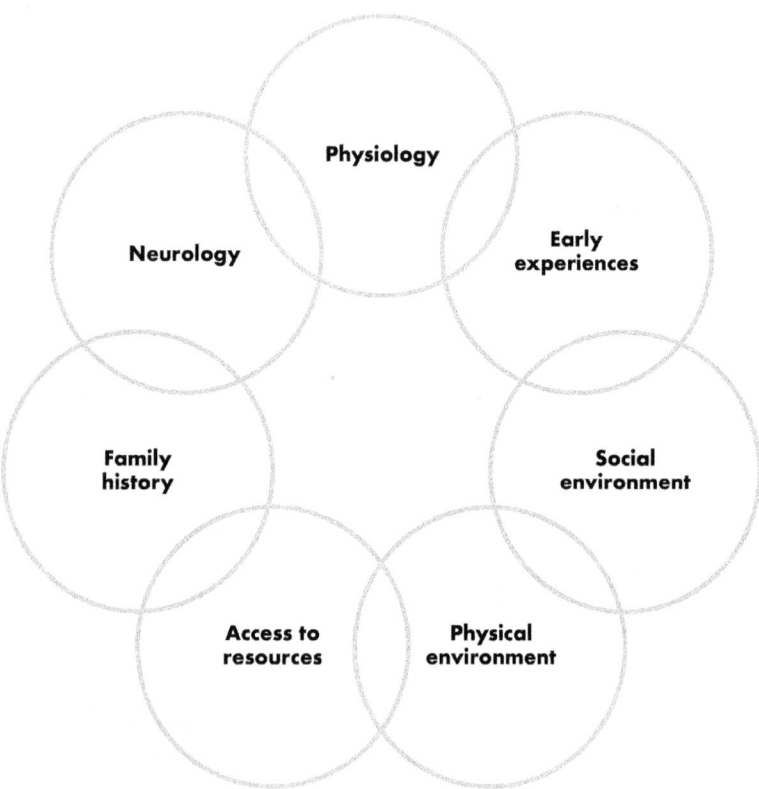

Figure 2.5 Factors that can impact speech, language, and communication development

Understandably, people are often looking for an explanation of why a child is finding things difficult.

Speech, language, and communication development is impacted by a range of factors:

- social environment (the people you grow up around, how people interact with you according to existing systems and structures),

- features of the physical environment, such as background noise
- physiology (the physical structure of all the body parts involved in talking)
- early experiences (attachment to caregivers, adversity)
- family history (whether other people in the child's family have/had any learning or communication difficulties)
- access to resources (if you're in an environment where people are struggling to have their basic needs met – things such as safety, food, shelter – then there can be less time and energy, and fewer funds for enriching experiences)
- neurology (differences in how brains process and respond to information)

While we may consider the variety of factors involved in how children develop communication skills, it's important to emphasise: *This is no one's fault.*

A big focus of communication support in the early years is around helping the caregivers to develop expert interaction skills that boost their child's progress. If you're one of those caregivers receiving that support it's not to say that you were 'doing it wrong' and caused your child's difficulties.

Lots of kids develop speech, language, and communication skills without an expert communication partner. You might even have older kids, or kids you've worked with, who developed these skills just fine. So, try not to blame yourself. And if you feel like blaming yourself, tell someone you trust. Talk it through together. I bet they'll reassure you emphatically that this is absolutely not your fault. Some kids just need extra help with this and that's what we're here to work on together.

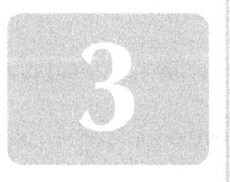

Build relationships

Include everyone from the beginning

Years ago, part of my job involved driving across the county and delivering speech and language workshops to early years practitioners (EYPs). At the end of each series, I would always deliver a workshop called 'Working With Parents'. It made sense to me at the time: focus on the child first, do some things to help them, then share that with carers so they can apply the same strategies at home. But, with this format, there's a risk of suggesting that some of us are the experts with all the answers, when, in reality, we have a lot to learn from each other.

Whether auntie, EYP, parent, speech therapist, or other, everyone who has regular contact with a child has an important perspective to contribute. So much of communication is experimenting and learning as we go along that we have to work a lot of it out together.

If we're to truly understand each child, we need the full picture of their everyday experiences and interactions: the things they love, the things they're familiar with, the things they like to talk about. How can we know what world we're imagining together, if we don't have some shared reference points? The favourite TV catchphrases, their routine at the park, the tune they hum when they put on their shoes. The food eaten, the festivals celebrated, the weekly cadence of a week. The more we know about a child's world, the more meaning we can notice and attribute to our interactions together.

R was a lad I worked with who would come to visit me with his mum. In our play together, he would position me in certain points around the room, while he made different sound effects and big actions (jumping, stretching,

DOI: 10.4324/9781003301967-3

falling to the floor.) I tried to join in, by observing what he was doing and copying or following actions occasionally, but it clearly had more meaning to him that it did to me. When his mum volunteered the fact that R loves *Jurassic Park* and will often fast forward to particular favourite scenes in the movie, my understanding of his play shifted. In discussion with mum, I saw how he was acting out the scene where the raptors chase the truck. His play included dinosaur sound effects, and some specific lines from the movie that I was only able to tune in to once his mum told me the details.

Same goes for M. He had a favourite song, '8 Planets of the Solar System' that he would often sing, or quote snippets from. Knowing the details of the song, as explained to me by his mum, helped me to recognise the details of what he was doing and join in with a more informed guess.

I sometimes find that parents are embarrassed to share these details, like they're not important or don't count as proper language. But they are, in fact, a hugely important part of the child's emerging communication. These are the things that are interesting and worthy of repetition. When we understand this perspective, we can tune in and respond to the details. We've established an important foundation for our interactions together: meeting the child where they're at, showing them that their interests and ideas are valuable, and that they can share them successfully with the people around them. This is how we all communicate and learn.

When we share the details, there's more chance of the child getting helpful repetition and consistency from a communication partner: play routines that become familiar and understandable across contexts, favourite phrases we can all use for common routines.

Parents might need a nudge to value and share these details of the sounds and word attempts that their child is making. Sometimes, these can be overlooked; it might be hard to attribute meaning to them without knowing more of their everyday environment and their cultural reference points.

The things that carers point out to me, their interpretations of a child's behaviour, are so important. We need every perspective. When we interpret something differently, we can dig into why and learn from each other.

Communication skills are built together. In the process of helping a child develop theirs, we're also developing our own. We're learning to tune in to the unique child in front of us: what's helpful to them and what helps our interactions be more successful. We're also developing our ability to reflect and talk about the details with other adults. Our communication skills even extend to learning to advocate for what a child needs.

We're raising this topic early in the book because I invite you to consider as you read:

- What ideas stand out for you and who do you want to share them with?
- What conversations would you like to have and with whom?

Let's start by valuing everyone's input. I want to hear what each person finds successful or fun about communicating with a child, so we can incorporate more of that into our plans and routines. We only ever get anywhere by sharing ideas and grappling with the mess together.

Aim for a flat hierarchy

With the various labels we're all given, it's easy to start looking for the 'expert', i.e., who's at the 'top of the list' for knowing the 'most stuff'. This type of hierarchical thinking puts us all at a disadvantage. It undermines our ability to learn from one another and work collaboratively.

Hierarchical thinking might suggest that the person with a title such as Speech and Language Therapist must be the 'holder of the information' and must impart their knowledge to everyone else. In this scenario, we're all at a disadvantage: the professional feeling the pressure to have all the answers, and the carer feeling the pressure to say the right things and not challenge. This dynamic doesn't result in the honesty and openness that we need if we're to try new things and make progress together. We lose the freedom to challenge and change. We set up a power dynamic that doesn't encourage open and honest conversation. It's far harder to ask searching questions of someone who arrives with 'all the answers' to the thing that you feel like you're failing at.

I love it when carers ask me questions, when they speak up in moments where I've said something confusing, or they have doubts about how my suggestions will work in their own family routine. I don't want to leave a therapy session thinking I've delivered important information, while the carer leaves thinking they don't know what to do or disagree with what I suggested. These moments of challenge give us the opportunity to develop our understanding together and come to tailor-made plans that make the biggest difference. So, we need to do what we can to welcome them, to establish a flat hierarchy where every contribution is valued.

Hierarchy doesn't just come from a professional label. There are power dynamics at play in all our interactions, based on various aspects of social identity. We may be aware of some of these, and we may be unaware of others. The 'Social GRACES' (Burnham, 2013) is a helpful framework for considering the many colliding aspects of our individual identities, and brings into consciousness considerations around how this impacts assumptions and privilege.

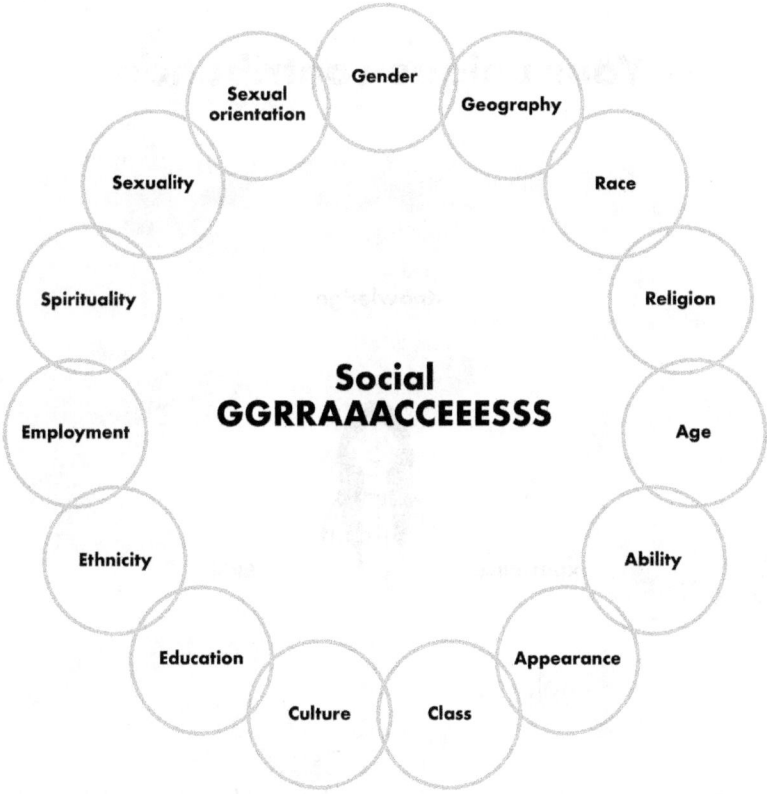

Figure 3.1 The Social GGRRAAACCEEESSS, Burnham et al.

When I lay out my own identity according to this framework (cisgender, British, White, middle-aged, middle-class, educated), it highlights the level of privilege, and therefore power, that I hold in many aspects of my identity. Being aware of this power and privilege is an important first step if we're to create relationships of safety, trust, and mutual respect.

Holding a position of power, asked for or not, is a great responsibility. In a role that involves coaching and supporting caregivers, we can impact how others *feel* about themselves and their capacity for change and contribution.

When we value contributions, we encourage more of the important details. We hear the important questions and points of challenge, our suggestions land as an invitation to explore, rather than a criticism or judgement.

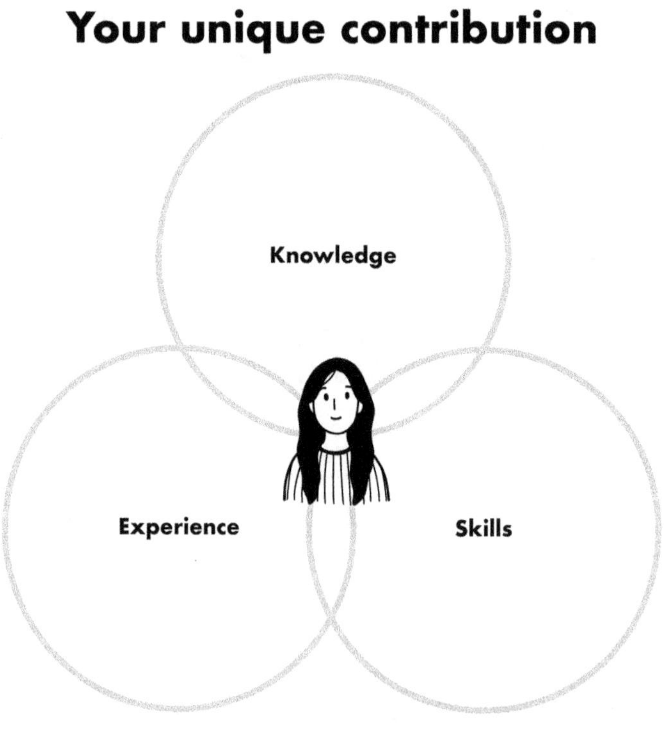

Your unique contribution

Figure 3.2 You bring your own particular blend of knowledge, skills, and experience to your interactions

That's not to say that we all hold the same information. We bring differing elements to our discussions together. As a Speech and Language Therapist (SaLT), I bring a detailed perspective and experience on communication development. In the background of my interactions with children, I'm noticing their processing speed, the pattern of their shifting attention, the gestures and sounds they form, and oh so much more. Then, I'm also factoring this into how I respond: what to focus on, how much or how little to contribute, when to pause, when to dive in etc.

I'm also considering the details of how the interactions unfold between caregiver and child: what each responds to, what points of connection seem successful, what opportunities we can build on together. Plus, I'm bringing along my experience of interacting with a whole bunch of kids with communication needs, coaching parents, having helpful conversations, and presenting information.

But still, *none* of this makes me an expert. I've got relevant skills and experience that bring value, and so have you. The experiences you've had, the skills you've gained, and the knowledge you've acquired are a rich tapestry unique to you, and we want to hear your thoughts!

So, instead of relating through hierarchy, we must relate through collaboration:

- What ideas do we hold together?
- Have we heard from everyone?
- Whose perspective have we overlooked through our own default assumptions?

We need to be able to share observations together, wonder out loud, challenge assumptions, question understanding, invite input from everyone in the room.

We need to ask caregivers:

- How do our observations compare with what you're seeing at home?
- What feels successful at home?
- What can we can learn from what you're already doing?
- How can we make the most of our collective expertise?

> REFLECT: What ideas do you have about who's in charge of communication? Do you have a sense of there being an expert that you must defer to, or are expected to be yourself? What are the power balances at play and how might this influence things?

These moments of openness and challenge are the moments that take courage and vulnerability. They're the moments where change is possible. We need to create an environment of safety that makes that possible. This starts with listening and staying out of judgement.

Practise active listening

In the early days of my career, I stuck closely to the script. I would ask carers the questions on the case history form, make sure all the boxes were filled in, and then dive into assessment and advice. What I didn't allow for was *time* – time spent listening to the things the carer wanted to tell me about their child. I didn't realise its value and it felt like there was never enough time.

It can be hard to prioritise this kind of time to listen when we're in work that centres around support for the child. But if we want to support the child, we must also support the carer. I'm in this work because I want children to feel heard and understood. That has to start with giving the carers the same opportunity.

When we give carers time to share all that's on their mind about their child's development, it can feel like we're not getting to the 'real work' of seeing the child. But the time that you give to listen to a carer is never wasted. It can only improve your relationship with the family and your insight into their communication ecosystem. We must take the time to listen and understand. We can't fast track this stuff.

I'm not a parent myself and this used to give me all kinds of feelings of inadequacy in my work. How could I possibly advise parents on this stuff if I didn't know what it was like for them every day? Over time I realised that being a parent wouldn't make me know what it's like for the family in front of me, because every family is different. I started to consider myself good enough. I thought about how I was the therapist they have. I might not be perfect at everything, but I was the one building a therapeutic relationship with the family. So I focused on staying present, willing to make suggestions and learn together.

My awareness of the contrast in our lived experience caused me to really prioritise listening. The only way I could hope to understand their situation was to ask and listen deeply to the answers. I couldn't assume that their experience was like mine.

This often means asking open and curious questions like 'How is that for you?,' 'Can you tell me more about what that looks like?,' 'What do you need from me?'

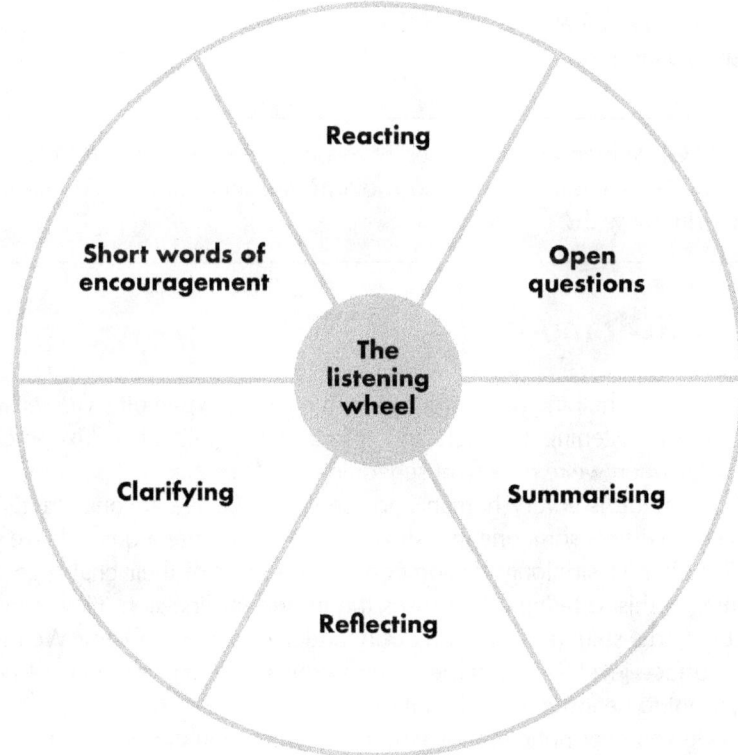

Figure 3.3 The Listening Wheel, illustrating a variety of possible responses when listening to someone

Source: © Samaritans 2005

Going beyond the specific questions in a case history form gives space for important information:

- What's going well?
- When do you feel most connected to your child?
- What's been helpful?
- What are you worried about?
- What would you like from me?

I find the 'listening wheel' from the Samaritans (Figure 3.3) a helpful reminder of the many varied ways in which we can enquire and respond to people, that makes them feel heard, and helps us listen to better understand their unique situation.

> REFLECT: Which of these types of response do you use most often? Which ones could you try more often? Are there any you'd like to experiment with?

Avoid fix-it mode

When we're in helping professions and labelled as experts it's very easy to skip over the 'listening to understand' part and get straight into 'fix-it mode'. Especially when we're on a tight schedule.

Fix-it mode is a very human impulse when we see anyone struggling. It's hard to witness someone in distress. It's easier to offer a quick 'Have you tried …', than to sit alongside someone in the mess of their challenge. But the thing is this: offering a fix misses the important first step. How can we possibly find a solution if we don't truly understand the problem? We might give a surface-level fix and in the process convey to the parent that we don't really want to hear the real difficulties.

Have you ever noticed those moments when you give someone a suggestion and it kind of stalls the conversation? The other person will say 'Yeah, I've tried that', or something else similarly vague, and it takes them out of the details of what they were describing. When we jump in with a solution, no matter how spot on we may be, it gives the message that we don't really want to hear the unique details of this person's situation. They start defending their actions so far, rather than telling you their insights hard won.

When we work with kids for many years, our brains naturally start sorting into broad categories, or take shortcuts and predictions towards what this child may need, because they fit into this broad group of descriptors in this way. It's simply what our brains do: shortcuts and predictions. So, of course, we often have a strong impulse to give suggestions and advice; we feel like we've seen this before and know what to do!

Knowing that we have this impulse to generalise and group is another reason to focus on listening to understand, rather than listening to fix.

When we have the opportunity to talk through the details, we're in a far better position to work towards a solution together, as our understanding grows.

> TRY IT OUT: Find a partner willing to practice active listening with you. You could share the listening wheel with them and explain what you're aiming to practice. Perhaps agree to take it in turns to be the listener. Set a timer and focus on listening to understand, rather than listening to fix.
>
> As you listen, try to use a variety of different listening responses, as illustrated in the listening wheel.
>
> Afterwards, ask your partner what they noticed about the exercise. What was their experience? What responses did they find helpful or unexpected?

Listening to genuinely understand can feel slow. It requires longer pauses, allowing for someone to say everything, giving time for us to formulate a considered response. This is a challenge if your listening time is a few minutes seized during pick-up or drop-off time, or a brief stay and play session.

Anticipate that challenge, the pull to be moving faster, to have got through the conversation faster. Plan for how you can allow more time. Perhaps change the time that you schedule meetings, or put less on the agenda, make listening to the carer an active goal in itself because everything else of benefit stems from this.

When you're listening, pay attention to your breathing. As a way to not run away with your own thoughts about what you should say next. Pay attention to how your body feels. I had a rude awakening when I was looking back on some video clips of a SaLT session – my shoulders were so tight and raised, my grin so wide. At the time, I had thought I was conveying to the carer 'I'm here, I'm listening', but my body looked like I was stressed and impatient.

> We're all communicating through our bodies alongside our words. So, can you be aware of your own body while you listen? Do you notice your thoughts running in other directions, in anticipation of how you'll reply? Can you really focus on attending to what the carer has said without planning the next step?

When we listen, we're a lot more likely to encounter the feelings that come along with the challenges of communication difficulties. And this is part of our work in the early years. When navigating a child's communication difficulties, and the responses from others around them, parents might be feeling lost, confused, determined, angry, hopeful, and more.

We can't detach these feelings from the work of helping the child to learn. Because, our own feelings impact our interactions: what we do or don't pay attention, what intentions we bring. We can help carers to tune into themselves, allow time for them to share their feelings and concerns. By listening and allowing for what parents need to share, we start to build a professional relationship, based on empathy and trust.

Stay out of judgement

While we might boldly say 'I don't care what people think of me', it's pretty hard not to care, maybe just a bit. We're social beings and feeling accepted by the group is a long-standing part of how we've evolved to work and live in community.

Our words, actions, and choices can be judged at any moment. People might think what we do is not enough, too much, inappropriate, or just plain wrong. It's tempting to defend ourselves when we feel this, to justify our choices, or argue with the other person's perspective. Judgements don't help us change, they lock us into defence mode.

At times, we all act from a place of defence, for fear of being judged. Perhaps we can use this insight, to gain perspective on how a parent might experience some types of support as judgement.

Sometimes, I wonder how much of parenthood is an exercise in being judged. On the bus, at the shop, strangers freely share opinions about what a child is doing, and how a carer is responding. Somehow, as observer, they think they know what's best for someone and what should be happening. No wonder parents can fear they're 'doing it wrong' or 'should know that already'.

I'm not a fan of the word 'should'. In fact, if you catch me in a crabby moment, I might even say that it's harmful. It sets a bar of expectation that so quickly sends us into a tailspin of panic over not doing *enough*. We blame ourselves or go into instant defence mode or feel immediately defeated and hopeless. Whichever way you view it, a 'should' doesn't inspire action.

What if we aim for interactions that are completely accepting of where they're at? We can start by acknowledging what they're currently able to do and willing to spend time with them to figure out what's doable for them. We understand one another better when we start from a perspective of respect, and an awareness that there may be many ways in which our differences affect our experiences and a wholehearted acknowledgement of the ways in which things may be hard for them.

We all have different levels of resources that impact our ability to act; differing levels of support and privilege, past stories, and challenges. Rather than assuming that a parent is somehow just *not trying hard enough* to help their child, I want to remember how much is unspoken, how much of their struggle I can't know. It's not always possible to read books at bedtime if you're working numerous jobs. It's not easy to remain calm and well-regulated if you have a history of trauma and abuse. It's a lot harder to successfully advocate for your child's needs if you're from a historically marginalised group.

We are living and working within a system that would have us blame the individual for these things. We can't change that in the short term, but we can approach people with love and understanding. We can start from the position that understands that everyone is trying their best and listen deeply to understand better.

Realise our shared humanity

I find it much easier to be understanding towards others than to myself. While I can acknowledge that everyone is trying their best and doing what they can with what they have, I still expect more of myself. I can't tell you the number of times I've thumped myself internally for not doing more or not being better.

The more I listen to others, the more I realise this is a common phenomenon. We all agonise over not being good enough, not doing enough for the kids we care for, or fear that someone else could do a better job.

> REFLECT: Write down your biggest fears about the work you do. What are you afraid people will realise about you or judge you for?

When I acknowledge how much I can struggle with this stuff, I start to get a glimpse of some of the fears a carer may hold. I fear letting a family down in a one-hour appointment. Imagine how a carer might feel if they are worried about letting their child down the whole time. Realising we can share these fears at times is an opportunity to expand our empathy and compassion. We're all muddling through; we can care for one another along the way.

The reality is that we're all juggling a lot and the moments that we have with a child, working on communication together, may not be 'optimal'. But they are what we have and checking in with ourselves is part of how we make the most of that time together.

So, take a breath and consider how you're feeling. Are you feeling wired and irritable? Or perhaps exhausted and low energy? Noticing and naming it is not only great modelling for our kids, it's also the first step towards better regulation. I believe that part of our role as speech and language therapists is supporting carers in this co-regulation. By being in the room with them, we are contributing to the emotional weather. Let's aim for smoother seas.

I had a conversation recently with the mum of a child I worked with when he was two and a half. The mum told me how those early interactions have flavoured her ongoing interactions with her son, who is now a teenager. I told her how uncomfortable I felt at the time, asking her to allocate some dedicated time to supporting his communication, when I knew how busy she was. She replied that actually the very routine of speech therapy sessions had created the space for her to regulate and spend the quiet, attentive quality time with her son that they both needed. It was a reminder for me of the fact that my own emotional state, regulated or not, impacts the feeling in the room, our ability collectively to settle down, and tune into one another.

'Celebrate with me'

This quote comes directly from a mum I worked with. She knew the difficulties for her child, she saw the contrast between him and his peers in nursery. She told me that the various professionals who visited spent all their time explaining to her in detail how we wasn't where he 'should be'.

In many ways, this is what is expected of professionals. The health visitors are required to carry out the two-year check, the speech therapists are required to assess and diagnose, the early years practitioners judge against age expectations.

This mum knew there was a long road ahead. She didn't think 'give it time and he'll catch up'. But she also wanted to talk about the things she was noticing, the moments that she wanted to celebrate.

I encourage you to value the moments of appreciation and celebration as much as your skills in assessment and analysis. We need to give carers the space to share the things that delight them about their child.

If a child is interacting and behaving in a way that many everyday people would judge as 'not right', then we may be some of the only people who can give the carer a different experience of being seen with their child. An experience of acceptance and celebration.

We must shift the narrative away from 'your kid's broken'. I meet carers who are in fight mode as a result of this narrative. How do you relax into a quiet moment of attunement with your child if you're fed so many stories of your child's strangeness, such tales of their lacking?

I don't want to be overly rosy about the genuine challenges for children developing differently. We need to be clear about what we're seeing, what this might mean for their development, and what support they may need.

There's a time for different modes: the quantified, standard scores that are required within our education system and the qualitative elements of care and attention that give carers a sense of hope and ability to act.

A speech therapist once told me that we're in the business of shattering dreams. Perhaps it's not about shattering dreams, but holding space while the ground shifts. Help me imagine a different future. Help me still celebrate my child. Because they are so truly worth celebrating.

Let's look at how we might do that.

Reference

Burnham, J. (2013) Developments in Social GGRRAAACCEEESSS: visible-invisible, voiced-unvoiced. In I. Krause (Ed.), *Culture and Reflexivity in Systemic Psychotherapy: Mutual Perspectives.* London: Karnac.

Start from strength

Tell a story of hope

When we talk about a child, we're developing a story about who they are and what they're capable of. We have choices about whether we tell a story of hope or of failure. The difference between the two is one of action and attention, over disappointment and exasperation. None of us can hope to try tricky things if we sense that it's 'no use'.

When it comes to surfing, I could be thinking about how I started learning too late, about all the past injuries that make it harder for me to learn. But, instead, I'm zoning in on how exhilarating it feels to be in the water, a vivid memory of that time I caught a crisp green wave early morning with no one else around. I'm thinking about how I can now pretty reliably pop up on the board (i.e., a tiny step). The way that it makes me grin so much of the time. Even knowing I may never be 'good', I'm so happy to keep trying and know that with practice and a positive mindset, I'll keep improving.

I aim to take this approach in all my interactions with the kids I meet. No matter how they're communicating right now, how different that may be from the majority, I want to approach every interaction with delight and appreciation for where they're at. I want to talk in ways that acknowledge the joy in the process and the ongoing tiny steps of progress I see along the way, knowing that this may be where we're at for a while, or that their progress over time may look different from that of their peers.

I appreciate it's easier for me to do this. In contrast to the parent learning about their young child, I'm calling on years of experience in interacting with children like theirs and seeing them develop. This makes it easier for me to believe in the value of what we're doing and the potential for progress.

DOI: 10.4324/9781003301967-4

I can't predict the future for any child, but I do have experience to inform my imaginings. I've been doing this work long enough to see kids grow into teenagers and to learn about their individual communication development. This isn't an evidence base in the formal sense. Instead, it's more of an imaginings base.

When I met R, I couldn't imagine that he would ever talk. It felt hard to connect with how he was experiencing the world around him. It was hard to predict how he would react to the things that I did. His mum and I judged our success in the early days by how long he was willing to stay in the room with us. Thanks to video clips and conversations by email and phone after our sessions, his mum and I learned to understand what was working for R: the ways he was communicating with us and the responses we made that he liked and that helped us build some back-and-forth interactions. Having seen him grow over the years and now hearing how he uses language and communicates with those around him gives me something to imagine for other kids.

It's often a matter of where we put our attention. Cognitive psychology teaches us that the story we tell ourselves about the situation, and what we notice as a result, impacts our mood and our behaviour. In a knock-on effect, our mood impacts how we interact. So we must prioritise helping a carer feel good about what's happening, about what they're seeing and doing with their child.

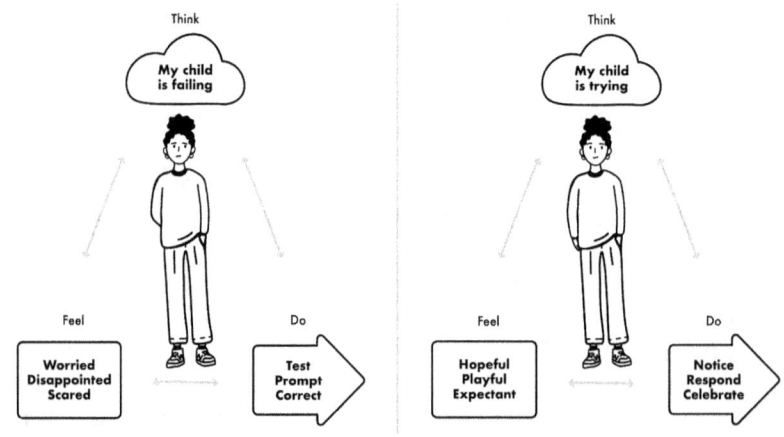

Figure 4.1 The story we tell impacts the way we feel and the way we approach things

Within an early years system that provides a whole gamut of tracking systems and monitoring charts, it can be hard to tell a hopeful story. What if your child is already 'failing the test'? Our early years systems are set up to identify need from an early age. We have our health visitors carrying out the two-year check, to identify children who are not meeting age-expected skills and an early education system that focuses on recording and tracking a child's progress from now until adulthood.

This creates a challenge for us: How to celebrate a child's unique communication profile, while acknowledging the extent of their support needs. How to be fully accepting of a child's attempts within a system that has clearly laid out expectations from the get-go.

We need both: 1) the measure of difficulties in order to plan for support, and 2) the celebration of a child in order to feel able to move forward. The way we talk about a child informs our ability to do this.

Let's look at two contrasting stories.

Trad Version

Billy's mum, Edith, knew something wasn't right from the beginning.

He didn't meet his milestones and the health visitor raised concerns. On the development charts, Billy was highlighted as 'all in the red'.

Edith was given several forms to fill, to get Billy referred to various professional services. The wait was agonising.

In the meantime, she researched everything online – what he should be doing, what she should be doing. It was scary because there's a lot of stuff online.

Edith worried that she had caused it and she felt the pressure to fix it. She tried to do the things the internet told her, but Billy didn't want to play ball and the two of them ended up frustrated and feeling like failures.

Alt Version

Billy's mum knew something was different right from the beginning.

He didn't seem to do the same things as the kids around him. Edith and her health visitor discussed this together. They talked about the kind of developing skills we look out for and what Billy might be doing differently.

Edith agreed it would be helpful to have extra support, to navigate the things that were proving tricky, and to better understand Billy's development.

In the meantime, Edith connected with a local group and reached out to friends. No one had all the answers, but they listened to her, and spent time with Billy.

Edith worried about the future because it was hard to know what to expect. But she and Billy had a growing support network of people who listened and showed her ideas that helped their play together. They had fun and celebrated the small wins. With the love and support of the people around her, celebrating what he was doing, and pointing out all the ways she was helping him, she didn't feel alone.

The story we tell about someone impacts how we approach them, what we expect, and what we leave space for. If we believe that a child is able to communicate ideas, even if they aren't talking, then we look out for those moments. We spend time with them looking out for the details. If we don't expect communication, or only value spoken words, then we can't notice and build on what they're doing.

We need to help parents tell a story of hope about their child, to notice and encourage the positive steps a child is taking in their communication however small. We need to help parents see and value the helpful things they're doing for their child. We all face an inner critic that can tell us we're not doing enough, and part of our role can be to help quieten those fears. This is what helps us to keep turning up and trying, even when it feels hard.

Describe what the child can do

When we describe the details of what a child is currently doing to communicate we help people to tune in and respond to these small attempts. In turn, this creates a positive feedback loop for the child: more experiences of successful interactions to learn from and build on.

With public services under-resourced and overstretched, there can be a need to emphasise a child's difficulties in order for their level of support needs to be acted on. But in the very early years, it should be less about campaigning for support needs by emphasising the child's failings, and more about describing to the parent what the child can do and helping them see the potential for change.

When I meet a child and am starting to build a picture of their communication profile these are the things I'm looking for:

- what they're paying attention to
- how they move their body, if there's anything I can interpret from their movements
- where they choose to be in the room (whether they approach people, if there's somewhere they appear to like to be)
- what objects/things/toys they're interacting with and how
- where they look
- what vocalisations they're making
- if they're coordinating any of these elements together (e.g., a gesture + a look + a sound)

Dr Dave Hewett, honorary life president of the Intensive Interaction Institute, summarised the 'Fundamentals of Communication', which are outlined below:

- enjoying being with another person
- developing the ability to attend to that person
- concentration and attention span
- learning to do sequences of activity with a person
- taking turns in exchanges of behaviour
- sharing personal space
- learning to regulate and control arousal levels
- using and understanding eye contact
- using and understanding facial expressions
- using and understanding other non-verbal communications
- using and understanding physical contacts
- vocalising and using vocalisations meaningfully (including speech)
- knowing that others care, learning to care

Attending to all of these details gives us information related to a child's communication. The little things a child does help us tap into their world, gain insight into their experience, which helps us support communication. The more that we can see the situation from the child's perspective, the more likely we are to spot the moments worth communicating about. It puts us in a better position to be able to join in with the child's play and follow, rather than lead (more on that in the next chapter).

So, first we notice and highlight the details of what the child can do. Then, we can discuss what might be next, the things that we might look out for. I meet many parents who are, understandably, looking out for *talking*. It's helpful to highlight all the other things that we might see a child do, to value, and therefore encourage all of the steps towards richer communication. For example, 'They're pointing now. Let's look out for whether they coordinate those gestures with a sound or a look.' Or, 'They're really interested in laying out their collection of dinosaurs. Let's pay close attention to the details, how it might change over time, and what sounds or gestures they might explore while they play.'

This level of detail requires video! We can only pay close attention to these things if we have a bit of time with the parent to slow down and revisit the play together. If we ask parents to pay close attention to such details in the moment, we get stuck analysing, instead of interacting with the child. You may well be much more practised at paying attention to these details and can do it 'on the fly'. The caregivers you support will need time to notice and value these details and imagine what might come next. When I share a video clip with a parent and pause or revisit a moment, they will often say 'I didn't notice that at the time!'

> PRACTICE: Thinking about your focus child, write a strength-based description of their communication. What are they currently doing and what might they be edging towards doing next? For this exercise, avoid any sentences that start with 'They can't…', or 'It's really hard for them to…'

Remember they're in the room

Have you ever had that feeling when someone is talking *about* you but not *to* you? It doesn't often happen to us as adults, because it feels rude or uncomfortable. We might even comment if it happens. ('I'm right here you know.') But we do this to kids all the time, particularly when they're not able to speak themselves. Conversations with carers about their children often happen while the child is in the room. Which is fine; we often talk about people while they're in the room. But only if we include them in it.

In any conversation about a child, I try to imagine that they can understand everything I'm saying about them, and also acknowledge them at times throughout the conversation. Kids pick up on a vibe.

Over the years, the more I think about this issue, it now feels uncomfortable to use a child's name and talk about them, while they're in the room. These days, I try to include lots of 'you' in my sentences; e.g., 'Charlotte, I notice you're trying out those /b/ and /d/ sounds. I see you looking and listening.' From there, the parents and I often go on to talk about the details. How we can respond to these sounds. What they've noticed at home etc. We do talk about the child while they're in the room, but we start by directing it at the child. This sets a tone of inclusivity, helps us remember to speak kindly, not critically, about what we see and where they're at.

> INVITATION: When you're in those conversations with parents and the child is in the room, try directing your starting sentences directly to the child, even if 'they're not listening'. Experiment with it and consider in what ways it changes how you and the parent talk things through.

Shift your language from disorder to difference

It can be tricky to speak in an accepting way about children, when much of the terminology of speech and language therapy is about lack or disorder. In the United States, our work is called speech and language *pathology*!

The language of disorder is baked into our profession, including many of the diagnostic labels we use: speech sound disorder, autism spectrum disorder, developmental language disorder. I use these labels, too, if the situation requires it; when a formal diagnosis informs other people of details, or facilitates access to services, or ensures acknowledgement of need for additional support.

Many of the kids I meet don't yet have a label or diagnosis. Those awaiting assessment for consideration of autism or ADHD can wait years. So, we have to continue to support without the label. This has given me the opportunity to get clear about what families need, what will make the biggest difference. It's helped me focus on each child's unique communication profile, rather than assuming I know them because they have a label. Yes, a label is helpful, but there's still lots we can do without it.

With or without a label, we can still consider the concept of neurodiversity in relation to the children we meet. This term refers to the differences in how brains process information. If we understand that different behaviours are not 'wrong', but instead may represent a difference in how a child processes, understands or interacts with the world, then this helps us to be more specific and non-judgemental in the language we use.

We're often required to compare a child against a prescribed set of data around what's typical for children as they develop. But when I'm thinking about and interacting with a child, this is not my primary frame. In fact, I'd argue that I don't need to think about 'what's typical' at all. I can focus instead on what they're doing and what's helpful. What makes them light up? When do they seem to be reaching out to me? What things do they respond to with joy or curiosity?

Instead of talking about what's wrong, or 'disordered', let's consider what's working and build on that. Using a frame of difference, rather than a disorder, doesn't mean we can't be truthful and direct about what a child finds difficult, but it does prompt us to talk with respect and acknowledgement of the fellow human in the room, however young they may be.

Respect at all times

In speech therapy, like many other health and care professions, our notes can be called on by anyone at any time. I've spent my career writing notes with an awareness that the client/individual may request access to them at any time. This has instilled in me a default position of clarity and respect, a desire to write notes without judgement, as objectively as possible.

It took longer for my verbal language match, for the things I said to be something that I would also say directly to the family. There's a risk of staff room 'real talk' (scare quotes intentional): shorthand assumptions or simplistic explanations of a complex family situation, which are different from what's said in conversation with parents. How can we hope to build an honest and trusting relationship with families, if the words we use about them are different when they're out of the room?

I'm grateful to the family support workers that I worked alongside in the past, who modelled an open and direct communication style. They were engaged in work that involved tricky, uncomfortable, and challenging conversations with families. They had to discuss care plans, removing children from harmful situations, and more. And, in all of this, they had a requirement to speak directly to the families about these matters. I found as a result that their own language in the office was respectful and considered. In their conversations between colleagues, they were taking the opportunity to practise using language they would also use directly with families.

When it comes to a child's communication and behaviour, we must use specific and accepting language about a child across all contexts, creating a culture of genuine appreciation and respect. The way we talk about a child affects our interactions with them. I don't need to give examples here. Simply consider: Would you be happy saying this in front of the family? Let's use our conversations with our colleagues as a way to practise open, clear, and non-judgemental language. Let's be genuine, authentic, and caring across all contexts.

Consider needs, not problems

It can be easy to get hooked on the problems. After all, that's usually the starting point for this whole discussion: Someone has flagged a child as not progressing like their peers. Then, an assessment typically involves judging the child against 'standard development'. My concern with this is that by focusing our attention on what they can't do, we leave little room for creating a positive story about the child and their potential.

One way that we can avoid lots of judgemental language around disorder and deficit is to focus not on what the child is *lacking*, but on what the child *needs*.

Perhaps they need:

- access to visual supports, to supplement their communication and support their understanding
- attuned adults who notice a child's communicative attempts and respond in a supportive way
- access to a space that is not overwhelming
- language spoken in short chunks, to aid their understanding
- time and opportunities to express themselves and develop new skills
- experiences of successful communication, in whatever form is available to them

The above is an incomplete list and these needs may change by context, age, and experience. It's intended as a starter; what would you add? Considering the child in front of you, what particular needs must be met in order for them to succeed? When we focus on need, we can shift away from what the child is failing to do or what they 'must do' in order to be deemed 'age appropriate'. Instead, we can focus on the adults, the environment, and the things we can do to support them.

> PRACTICE: Building on your written description of a child's strengths from earlier in this chapter, add to that a list of the things that you notice the child needs. Think about things that help the child to engage or be successful in getting their message across.

Trust in capacity

I always encourage parents to give their child the benefit of the doubt. If you think that maybe, just maybe, your child had a go at that word, then go with it! Think optimistically. Allow yourself to celebrate it, even with the possibility that you were just imagining it. When we think like this it puts us in a position of enthusiastic response. It increases the likelihood of responding in a way that encourages communication.

Assume that the sounds and actions your child is making as an attempt to connect and communicate with you. Assume that the things they find interesting are important. Assume that the way they choose to explore and play is right for them and is supporting their learning and development. When you start from that mindset you're more likely to respond in a way that supports further interaction between the two of you.

If they are lining up toys, or throwing things, or choosing to play with the door wedge instead of the toys, it can be tempting to jump to thoughts about this not being 'proper play' or a 'red flag' for disordered development. But, what would happen if you trust in the value of how the child is choosing to explore, and start from where they're at?

I visited a nursery once where the manager said to me: 'You won't get a response from him because you're not chalk.' This young boy loved chalk; he loved sorting the chalk by size and colour; he loved the way he could shake the chalk in the jar, and how he could draw big circles on the floor. (There's probably countless thing about the chalk that make it super-satisfying for this child, but, at the time, he didn't have the communication tools to tell us about all of that.) I think what the practitioner was trying to convey to me was that competing for the child's attention felt impossible when chalk was around: 'Chalk is exciting to this kid; there's no way you can be that exciting.' With this as the nursery's story, it was hard for the adults to connect with the child and vice versa. They saw him with the chalk and thought he was better off left alone with it. When they did try to interact with him, it was all about trying to pull his attention away from the chalk. So, this kid was experiencing a lot of his interactions as being pulled away from his favourite thing.

Part of this no doubt comes from the idea that we know what's best for a kid. That we should make an assessment of their learning and development and decide what the plan is, what they need more or less of. The common assessment I encounter (and have definitely made myself in the past) is that this kid needs to broaden their interests, that there's nothing to learn from chalk.

Instead, we could start from a place of trusting the child, and trusting in the value of their exploration. This child had a rich repertoire of different ways to explore the chalk. My challenge was to pay attention to the details, learn from him, be a willing and available partner to his play.

So, I sat alongside him and tried joining in with the chalk. I took my own piece of chalk and tried copying some of the things that the child was doing. Some of these things he appeared tolerant of and some he told me to stop, by taking my item or vocalising that he was unimpressed. Absolutely fine by me. I didn't try to insist on my plan. After all, play is about experimenting. I didn't need to be right. And I was glad when he told me that what I was doing didn't work for him. My goal was to learn what was fun about the chalk, to find out if it was possible to join in and share chalk appreciation together.

Over time, I learned the way to play with chalk that the child enjoyed. He was interested when I drew large circles on the floor. He watched when I filled my own container with chalks, while he did the same with his. These small things over time communicated to the child that we can have fun together, that an adult being near him didn't mean he had to stop his favourite thing. Instead, we could appreciate it together. I hope that he felt able to settle and engage, not in what I was teaching him, but in what we were exploring together. Each child I work with teaches me new perspectives, new ways to explore, new ways to be a part of their rich world. I don't want to miss that! Trust in the value of what the child can show you.

Let the child lead

Tune in to the child's point of interest

Do you remember that feeling as a kid when the smallest things were absolutely fascinating? At that age, everything is new and worth exploring. I'm not sure I remember those moments specifically, but I have a sense memory of it when I see the deep fascination and delight in the way kids explore. The way they squat down to examine a piece of gravel or stop in their tracks to figure out the source of some certain sound.

When they're drawn to the water tray and want to splash the trucks on the surface, it's hard for me to suggest that I might have a better plan. Because for that child, just imagine how exciting that is!

If the child is really engaged in the hydrodynamics of splashing trucks, then their capacity to learn is strong. By starting from that existing spark of interest, we're much more likely to facilitate the child's potential for communication.

Establishing enjoyment together and sharing ideas isn't achieved by my pulling the child away from their chosen activity, but instead by taking note of their interest, helping that child to learn that their ideas matter to me and I'm available for all the variety of things they might like to share.

Our initial goal is always to establish some shared enjoyment. It's easier for us to do that by joining in with the child's choice, rather than suggesting an alternative.

As a first step, I want the child to realise they can invite me into their play by communicating their ideas. Ideas that might be something like, 'Let's do this', or 'Cool sound!', or 'No, not like that!', or 'Stop!'. All ideas that can be conveyed without needing words. I want to build on their capacity to lead me, rather than their capacity to follow my lead. Because communication is about unprompted spontaneous shared moments.

Communication becomes intrinsically rewarding when it helps us share plans. When I first meet a kid, I want them to learn the joy of sharing their ideas, seeing that I will follow them. I want to find out what the child's plan is and to find a way to be a part of it that still feels comfortable for the child. I'm looking for something shared that we can build on.

My most effective way of doing this is to pay attention to what they're already doing and over time look for opportunities to respond and join in. This often starts by sitting alongside.

I had a recent first session with a child, sitting alongside while he lined the cars up in front of the TV, then moved them one by one to the toy microwave and then down to the toy sink. After a while I tried passing the child one of the cars to put in the microwave. He accepted and put the car in the microwave along with the rest of them. Over time, this simple sequence developed between the two of us. The child passed me items, we started putting the cars in other places, we started adding other things to the microwave.

I describe this as sitting alongside in order to emphasise the fact that you don't have to be doing or directing in any way. Instead, it's about tuning in and responding. It's about communicating to your child that you are totally interested in how they see the world, that you're curious and want to join in with what they're doing.

Sitting alongside might look like:

Waiting and watching. Giving yourself time to notice the details of what's interesting for the child, to notice their point of attention, observe their actions, and hear their sounds.

Reflecting what you see and hear. Making the same sounds, doing the same actions/gestures as your child as a 'reply'.

Not expecting a response. Reflecting and replying without wanting anything from the child.

Accepting a slow pace or 'not much happening'. This acceptance without expectation of things progressing in a certain way is crucial to following a child's lead. It stops us from prompting or trying to move things on. It leaves us available to notice and respond to what the child is doing.

Joining in with a toy or action. Picking up something similar to what the child has and playing in a similar way alongside, or handing the item to the child.

Keeping chat to a minimum. When we talk a lot, we're at risk of dominating the airtime and leaning towards director mode. When we say less, we give space for the child to make more sounds, try new actions, invite us into their play.

We might hope to contribute our own ideas to the play, but getting to that point takes time and there's plenty of steps before that, so we mustn't rush in with our own preconceived plans. If that child has had lots of experiences of adults trying to change the play, then it can take time to build their trust that you won't change or 'mess up' their play plans. I often hear from parents that a child doesn't like it if they touch a toy or get too close to the play. This may well be because their common experience is that adults getting close means the play gets changed.

How frustrating this must be for the child who can't tell us their plan for the play. Perhaps their only option is to protest with a scream or a shove that says: 'Don't come too close, you'll mess it up!' One of the key things that I'm exploring when I spend time with a child, especially early on, is to find their comfort zone for me being a part of things.

Are they ok with my …

- sitting near them
- getting close to have a good look at what they're doing
- making sounds or gestures about what's happening
- handing a toy to them
- playing with another toy alongside them
- adding a toy to the play

This isn't presented as a formal hierarchy, more a smattering of things I try in the spirit of experimentation. As the child can't necessarily tell me what feels good for them, and I can't be certain they understand what I'm saying to them, we have only this gentle doing; trial and experimentation. Being able to communicate these things is a priority: what feels good, what feels interesting, what gets a 'yes', and what gets a 'no'.

Children with communication needs are at greater risk of harm as they grow up, so helping them to say no and learn that their 'no' is respected by those around them is essential.

By sitting alongside and not directing the play, the child learns they can say yes and no to our participation. Initially, practising communicating together, is about what they want and don't want, not about what I want.

This means that some of my speech therapy sessions finish early or change entirely.

If a child grabs his coat to indicate that he wants to leave the room, we can do that. I want them to know that their actions have an impact, that their behaviour communicates stuff that the adults respond to.

> OBSERVE: Spend some time watching your child's play, without trying to get too involved. Look for the details of what they're doing. What do you notice?

Give it space

One of the greatest challenges in supporting the steps of early communication is allowing ourselves to do less. It can feel counterintuitive to step back when we are so keen for our kids to move forward. We can quickly fill up all the airtime with commentary on what's happening.

When we do all this talking, try to grab their attention and teach them new words, two things can happen:

1 There becomes no need for the child to speak/act/communicate, because all the talk is being done by someone else.
2 The child can withdraw because the additional talk is adding to their processing load, easily overwhelming them when they're trying to focus on an important part of their play.

When we do and say less we create space for the child to do more, to take the lead and be in charge of how the play goes. This kind of quiet can feel genuinely uncomfortable for us and not 'enough', but it is actually vital thinking time for a child.

When I stop trying to get the child's attention I find I'm often waiting longer, but after a while the child will start to seek me out, look towards me for a response to what they're doing. A look that says 'Did you see that?', Or 'Where are you?'.

You might like to play around with this idea yourself. When you sit with your child, quietly attentive, rather than talking, what happens? At first, it may feel like 'not enough', and it will take time for both of you to readjust to a different pace and different rules. But it's worth the initial discomfort, to give your child the valuable space to explore how they want to lead, to think about what they want to communicate with you, and experiment with how they can do that.

> REFLECT: How does it feel for you to not be busy? Is the quiet uncomfortable or ok? By becoming more aware of how it feels to be less busy, we can avoid falling into busy on autopilot. What could you tell yourself in the moment to allow yourself to sit and be quietly present with your child?

Children need patience and expansive space to explore, test, discover, and learn. They often need us to attentively and quietly notice what they're doing and allow space for it to unfold, responding to what they do, rather than directing how we think it should go.

Keena Cummins, Speech and Language Therapist and founder of the 'VERVE Child Interaction' approach, encourages adults to wait for the child to look at you before you speak or act. This helps the adult focus on *responding*, by actively waiting for a cue from the child. If the child is comfortable with eye contact then this strategy can give the child agency over the *pace* of the interaction, how much is said, how quickly things move along. This agency reduces the risk of the child feeling overwhelmed by too much; all the talk or the busyness of the adult. You might view the moment when a child looks to you as an invitation, a moment when they are indicating: 'Your turn, what do you think?'

Look for the invitations

In video feedback sessions, I often point out 'invitations' that the child extends. When they pass you something, or hold something up to you, when they point and vocalise at something, inviting you to notice it.

These invitations can take time to emerge, sometimes weeks of practice. After all, if stepping back and giving space is a new strategy for you, it will take some time for the child to adjust, to learn that they can set the pace and make things happen. When we give space, we give the child time to learn that they have agency over how we play together.

It always makes me smile when a parent starts talking about invitations. They might point them out in a video of their child, or use the word when retelling an anecdote about their recent play together. We all love to receive an invitation. When kids aren't speaking, it can feel like a personal rejection, so understanding that these small acts of initiation from a child are a truly special thing can be a valuable way that our language shifts how we feel about things.

Directing vs. responding

Once we're tuned in to the child's perspective and the details of their play, we can look for ways to join in, to make it a shared activity full of opportunities for communication, while still letting them lead. Child-led play means a focus on *responding* to what the child is doing rather than *directing* how it should go, thinking we know what the child needs to do next in order to learn or be doing it 'properly'.

On the beach in the summertime, I often spot the Director Dads. I see them standing at the edge of the water, full of instructions. Their kids are splashing about in the water, or wobbling on a paddle board, or jumping into the waves. And I hear: 'Stand back', 'Be careful', 'Hold your arms out', 'Watch out for that person behind you.'

Why do they stand at the edge and direct instead of joining in? Is it fear, or reluctance, or exhaustion? Perhaps it's embarrassment or uncertainty? I suspect it's a complex mix of different (and totally valid) emotions. While I'm not the dad at the water's edge, I am sometimes that adult trying to manage from a distance, a little uncertain about my role and a little afraid of what might happen if I try to join in.

When we try to join in, without knowing where the play will go, we're more vulnerable to failure or criticism. This is why starting from strength is so important. We need to have a sufficient feeling of 'enough-ness' about ourselves to be willing to try. This stuff feels hard and scary, which makes it tempting to avoid. If you don't try, you can't fail.

Perhaps we direct because it feels more 'grown up'. As adults, our everyday lives are easily stripped of playfulness. Judgements are made about our performance, there's important stuff to do and we mustn't waste time being 'silly'. I'll always remember the guy I saw riding his kid's scooter home from the school run. When he saw me clock him, he quickly jumped off and started walking. Are we afraid of being seen as unserious?

I wonder if this seeps into our interactions with kids: the idea that we must take the play seriously, use it as a teachable moment rather than mess about and find genuine joyful connection. A dad I worked with recently told me that learning to follow his child's lead made the play more fun for him too. His child, Z, came up with more unexpected ideas than the concepts that Dad thought he should learn. When we watched back a video clip together we could see how Dad was aiming for the child to say how the toys live *next* to one another, but instead Z said 'double house'. Dad chuckled, repeated it back, and their play moved on together, Z jumping up and down with the excitement of it all.

Maybe we think that this business of learning is about trying hard and completing the correct sequence of steps. This mindset can make it genuinely challenging to follow the child's lead. If you follow them, respond to their plans, join in with their actions and sounds, I can guarantee there will be moments when you'll feel silly. That is almost the point. To let go of thinking about the future and what your child needs to learn and instead focus on the simple fun of being together.

Children with communication needs are at risk of being very directed. It's easy to get into director mode with someone who isn't saying much. Their pace may appear slower, their communication attempts smaller, so the supporting adults might naturally give more prompts, to pick up the pace, and get more of a sense that something is happening. Silence is awkward, and we fill the airtime with questions or instructions, simply so we don't have to sit quietly.

> REFLECT: If you work with a group of children, do you notice a difference in how directive you are with each one?
>
> What's more comfortable for you – directing the play or sitting alongside and responding to the child's invitations? How does this impact your child's experience? Have you noticed how your child responds to each mode?

But what about *modelling*?! Isn't that a way that we should direct and teach children?

Modelling is the act of us adults doing something that serves as an example that the child can learn from and use themselves. In pre-school, we often focus on modelling key words that are relevant to the activity. For example, if we were playing with the toy kitchen, we might have a plan to model making cups of tea and saying 'Pour it in', 'Have some tea', 'That's hot!', etc.

Modelling is important, and is a valuable part of how we support children. But let's not dive in with it too soon. The risk with modelling is that we dictate what's most important. We choose the words we think they should hear and copy, we take the lead by modelling the actions we think the play should include.

Modelling expects the child to already be attending to us and understanding the copying nature of communication. Modelling language and copying it is a key part of communication development and some kids simply do it. Others need a little more practice to learn the concept that listening and copying is part of what we do together.

If we prioritise modelling words and phrases before we've established a shared connection with the child, then we're simply throwing words into the room with little impact.

As the child starts to learn that we're responsive to them, they can start testing this out. They can try new actions or sounds, to see how we'll respond. We can be the communication whiteboard they can scribble on, to see their own actions and sounds reflected back. We can aim for everything they try out to get some kind of response from us; a simple cause and effect.

Until we've established with the child a reason for them to engage and attend to us, we have to prioritise what the child's already doing, tune in to them and respond to what they're doing, rather than expecting them to tune in to us and copy what we're modelling. Modelling doesn't *have* to be directive.

You can model language in a way that is still attuned to their interests and in *response* to what they do. In the next chapter, we'll talk more about choosing our moments and being *intentional* with the things we model.

Give attention to get attention

Attention is a funny thing. We all struggle with it at times, particularly when interacting with others. We also know how essential it is for learning. So it's understandable to ask: How do I get my child to pay attention to me? We think that this is the first step towards communication: 'If I could just get them to listen to me, then they could learn.' I'm not in disagreement with this. Attention is a hugely important part of learning. But, in these early stages, it's not about simply getting the child to pay attention to us. From their perspective, why should they? What you say is hard to interpret, what you do isn't as fun as their own plan, what you're asking them to do is tricky.

Attention development starts by being able to maintain focus on something the child finds inherently interesting, focusing on it without any encouragement or prompting. When we consider attention development, especially in early years settings, we move quickly to adult-led attention. But actually, there's still lots children gain by pursuing their own point of attention, without having to follow our lead.

Back to the cars in the microwave ... The child's mum commented that this was longer than he ever usually plays with one thing or with one person. I suggest that the reason he attended for longer and stayed in the play was because it was about *his* point of attention. We started from the thing that he found naturally intriguing, rather than by trying to pull him in a different direction, something that I might have judged to be more worthwhile.

It's no use our constantly prompting and performing to try to grab a kid's attention. Instead, we need to show them what quality attention looks like, by giving it to them without expectation, practising genuine prolonged focus and interest in what they're doing. If we want to *get* attention, first, we need to *give* attention. Simple, right? Not so much. There's myriad different things in our environment pulling on our attention. So, it can feel hard to give our full attention to a child whose play seems baffling to us and whose communication attempts are small. No wonder we try to grab their attention and pull them towards something *we* think is more interesting.

The practice is in tending to what *is*, right in this moment, rather than wanting something different. I want to see what happens when I give my attention to what's actually happening, rather than wondering what *should* happen next. If we are noticing the details of how a child is playing, rather than teaching them the 'next step', then we're in a better position to join in in a way that the child finds fun and worth engaging in.

Solutions for when it's hard

While we might all be in agreement about the benefit of following the child's lead it can be deceptively hard to actually do this. The ways that we pull children away from their own point of interest can be quite subtle. We might not even notice we're doing it.

We might feel simply too busy to go at the child's pace and let things unfold. We might feel the pressure to get on with getting stuff done.

Whatever your role, there's invariably a push for time, a sense that you've got more requirements being made of you than can possibly fit into the hours of the day. The sheer amount of stuff to do demands a busy pace; the kind that has you mentally prepping or ticking off the next thing on the list even while you're still doing the first. It's very easy for us to meet kids with this kind of energy. When we have things to get done, watching a child contemplate the intricacies of a tiny speck of fluff on the carpet doesn't feel easy. It's hard to feel patient about the time required to allow for a child's deep focus when there's so much else going on.

Children often don't fit with a busy schedule, unless we push and drive it. That busy forward motion works for plenty of things: getting kids to school on time, organising a bunch of kids around a regular snack schedule, making sure everyone takes a turn.

But this busy pace doesn't work if we're aiming to develop communication together. When our kids are learning to reach out and try different ways of communicating, these things can be subtle and small. They can also take a long time. This communication time can be full of long pauses, awkward silences, and the feeling that *nothing is happening*. And when you have a long to-do list, how do you square that? My suggestions are as follows:

Allow it to look like 'nothing'

It can be quite a mindset shift to trust that your attentive presence and willingness to respond, but not lead, is genuinely useful. That you are actually doing the work of supporting communication.

If you work in a busy early years setting, you may need to talk with your team about what you're trialling: 'It might look like I'm doing nothing.' This frees you from feeling the need to appear industrious. Because, while it might look small, you and that child are practising an essential interaction skill: attentive presence. We're tuning into the child's perspective on the world, the things that fascinate them. That might be:

- the way that the fire alarm beeps intermittently
- the play of light as you pour water into the tray
- the satisfying clunk of that cupboard that fits in the frame just so

Dedicating time at a slower, quieter pace is essential for our non-speaking kids. But it may pose a challenge within a busy setting. Talk as a team about what solutions there might be for this. Are there pockets in the day or week when things are a little less hectic, so that you can dedicate some time to going at this pace?

> PLAN: What are the parts in your daily/weekly routine where it may be possible to go at a slower pace, without being pulled in different directions or sticking to a schedule?

Regulate to communicate

We can all relate to times when we don't communicate effectively or don't even want to communicate because we feel down or stressed, overwhelmed or infuriated. Emotions are a huge part of the communication ecosystem. You can't truly connect when you're stressed.

Our own ability to be calm and attentive is a genuine part of the practice of developing communication together. The only way we can hope to be able to follow the details of a child's communication and respond in a helpful way is if we're attentive and available. (A note of realism here: I think there's plenty of times when we can turn up as just good enough and muddle through and still establish positive and supportive relationships with the child. But, if we are thinking about what puts the situation in our favour, then being well-regulated ourselves is genuinely of value.) What can you do to push things in the direction of feeling well-regulated yourself, acknowledging that you likely live and work within a bunch of forces that make it harder to be calm and attentive?

Our success in communicating together is impacted by our ability to regulate our energy and mood. That's part of why it's important to consider the whole family system in which the child is growing. We can't hope to support a child's communication if we're feeling fraught. The child can't hope to be successful if they're stressed or upset.

Children rely on us to help them regulate their mood and energy levels, so how we feel impacts this. You probably have a bunch of external pressures playing on your mind too; expectations, to-do lists, worries and tasks. All these things accumulate and affect how we connect and communicate with others. This is something we share with kids. The only difference is that their difficulties in regulating themselves may be more physically apparent, whereas we adults tend to sit still but be highly distracted internally.

This is not to say that if your child is having a hard time regulating that it's your fault. We're simply looking at the things that might nudge it in our favour.

> REFLECT: What are the things that make you feel stressed and distracted? List as many as possible. In that list, you may find some that you have some control over and can plan the reverse for the times when you want to optimise your communication time together.

Allow the play to look unexpected

It can also be hard to follow a child's lead if it feels they're not doing it 'properly'. We might feel the pull to help or teach, to get them to *do more*. We might want to show the child how they should be playing with the toy, to construct the train track so that it loops up 'properly'.

Part of the challenge of following a child's lead is noticing our own judgements about what their play should look like. It can take time to adjust to how this particular child chooses to explore and experiment with what's around them. Before we dub a child's play 'restricted/obsessive/non-constructive/repetitive' can we take a moment to consider how the child views the activity? What makes it interesting? What parts do they like to repeat and how does it subtly shift over time? By trusting the child's *own point of interest*, we shift our perspective to accept how they're exploring and get curious about the details.

You may have come across the stages of typical play development: exploratory, relational, symbolic, role play. Understanding these different types of play can help us tune in to what we're observing.

Not all children go through these in a neat sequence and one isn't better than the other. The danger with laying out stages like this is that we push for the next stage and don't value the child's own mode of discovery and fun in the moment. If we have a sense of what new skill they need to demonstrate, we risk interrupting the thing they're currently figuring out, or getting in the way of the communication or increased complexity/richness.

Play is fundamentally about exploration and curiosity. When we remember these basic principles, we can be more accepting of the many different ways children explore and what they gain from this. Play can look like: enjoying the look of something in the light, viewing it from different angles, moving your body in different ways, arranging things, making sounds, repeating things over and over for simple joy, experimentation, learning about consistency.

It's all play. Let's respect it and give it space to unfold.

Avoid the toy trap

Sometimes the work of early attention and engagement with someone else demands full focus. Noticing actions, attending to facial expressions, playing with sounds etc. All of that is enough to explore and learn from, without needing many toys.

I'm often asked for recommendations of toys that support language development and sure, I have got some favourites. But toys can be a distraction from the real work of being available and attuned to the child, allowing for their interest in playing chase, or bouncing on our knees or singing a song. All these everyday activities offer valuable communication practice and none involves a toy.

I've fallen into the toy trap countless times, trying to get the child's attention on a toy, or pull them from their point of attention to a different toy, because I feel that we should be 'moving on'. A shift happened for me when speaking with a colleague who asked why I was trying to get the child's attention on the toy when the child was clearly interested in my face. If we're helping with the early stages of communication, what could be more valuable than allowing for sustained interest in faces? Why did I imagine that the tambourine or the stacking cups would enrich that moment of attunement more than that child's spontaneous desire to explore my face?

When we prioritise toys in the play, we get hooked on commentary – lots of talk about the stuff, without space for the child to take a turn. I've been the adult who thinks that communication has to somehow be about *things*. The teddy or the train. Many kids do learn language through everyday chitchat about the things around us. But this type of commentary doesn't work for all children, especially the ones who need extra time to explore the foundational skills: attention, engagement, turn-taking. By all means, enjoy the toys, explore things together. But beware the moments when you're trying to get the child to pay attention to the object instead of allowing them to simply be with you.

6 Choose your focus

Decide what's important

> REFLECT: Think back to a time when you've had a really positive interaction with someone. Maybe a good heart-to-heart chat with a friend. Spend a minute sitting in the memory of that. What felt good about it?

Perhaps you felt like you were really heard and had the opportunity to clarify things by talking it through. Perhaps you were both fired up about the topic and sparked ideas together. Perhaps you felt like you really got to know the other person better. I like to start here so that we can tap into what we're aiming for when we support children. We may have concrete goals for the skills we hope to see develop in a child, but, first, how do we want our children to feel?

Taking on the advice of Magda Gerber, early childhood educator and founder of RIE (Resources for Infant Educators), I aim to view each child I meet as a unique human being who I can share space and ideas with. Just as I do in my approach to the parents and practitioners I work with, I want to create a sense of respect and appreciation. I don't want to make the mistake of thinking that I, as the adult, have all the answers and they are small empty vessels to be filled with my knowledge and expertise. Young children are so much more than that. Their own experiences, ideas, perspectives are all valuable and something that we can learn from, or certainly engage with openly. Don't fool yourself into thinking you always know best, or even that you're required to.

When I think back to some of the good conversations I've had, it's often been at times when I felt truly accepted, with all my wordy quirks and geeky enthusiasm. To have been heard and not judged. To have the sense that it's ok to be me and it's ok to say what's on my mind. It feels good to have conversations where there's space to hear what everyone's said and permission to be your full messy authentic self. Space that allows moments of pause between talk, a sense of comfortable quiet.

Certainly, not every conversation is like this. A lot of the time, I'm second guessing or overthinking, wondering if the other person is bored, or I've said too much, or done something terribly uncool or inappropriate. You too? Suffice to say, not all interactions go smoothly. That's part of living in community with others.

I think it's interesting how low-pressure situations can lead to the richest conversations. I'm thinking about those places and activities, like going for a walk with someone, or being in a knitting circle, where active conversation isn't expected the whole time. These situations can free people to think more deeply or speak more thoughtfully, without the pressure to fill an empty silence. I hope that we can create similar conditions for our kids: a space where there's no pressure to talk, but, instead, there is time to think and go slow, and a receptive ear is available when there is an idea to share.

Conversations feel good when we build on one another's ideas, when something said was really interesting and sparked a neighbouring idea. Things were funny and playful, words flying, mistakes embraced, random links made, silly voices tried on for size. Conversations don't have to be serious to be worth our time.

In a conversation full of spoken language, it's easy to see how we build ideas together. Perhaps you mention the weather forecast for the weekend, I might add to that by saying it'd be a good weekend for a picnic, you might agree and talk about your favourite picnic foods, it might be olives. I could add that I love the olives with the garlic cloves stuffed inside them, etc., etc. Conversation is a back-and-forth. When it's good, we're paying attention to one another's contribution and adding to it. (Quite different from the 'waiting for your turn to speak' style of conversation.)

In an interaction with a non-speaking child, we can still build on one another's ideas. The main distinction is that the ideas are very much in the present moment. They're about the environment we're in, the ways we can move our body, explore the things around us, and make sounds. These are all things that we can join in with and build on. A child's idea might be to bounce the superhero figures on the coffee table. I could build on that by adding my own figure to the coffee table. If we've been doing this a while, I might add something extra. A tumble turn or sound effect for that superhero figure. It doesn't matter *what* we're doing. It's the quality of our attention and acceptance for how the child is exploring and interacting with us.

Decide at the core what's most important to you about your interaction together. Is it getting them to say a new word, or is it about building your relationship together? Sometimes reminding ourselves of what we're here for can help us to value these exchanges even when we feel disappointed or worried about a specific detail.

A note on mindfulness

Have you ever sat and watched a bird that's just landed near you? Have you noticed how the feathers puff out in the wind, the way their head cocks to the side, the small movements of their beak and their feet as they settle on to their perch? As I sat down to start this chapter, just such a bird (a crow, actually) landed on a post outside my window. There's a certain kind of unobtrusive attentiveness required when watching other animals, somehow sitting in a way that doesn't cause them to dash off the moment they notice you.

Of course, the only reason I watched this bird in such detail was due to the procrastination that's inherent in writing. To sit and observe details without any outcome or end goal can feel like 'time wasted'. But actually, in these moments, we're practising something that is crucial for quality attention, conversations, and wellbeing. It's a valuable exercise for us humans, to stop and truly notice what's happening right now.

Mindfulness describes a state of quality attention and awareness of the present moment. The aim is to focus on what's happening right here and now, without ruminating on something that's already happened, or some plan for the future. As the wise tortoise in *Kung Fu Panda 2* reminds us: 'Yesterday is history, tomorrow is a mystery, but today is a gift. That is why it is called the present.'

While I love the wordplay of this quote, DreamWorks Animation didn't invent mindfulness. The historical roots of meditation date back thousands of years, linked to religions including Hinduism, Buddhism, and Judaism. There's a growing body of research on its benefits, including managing anxiety, depression, and stress. The reason I'm interested is because it can help us calm the mental chatter and be truly attentive to the child we're sharing space with. And that quality attention impacts the quality of our interaction.

I have plenty of moments through daily life where I am in the room, but my mind is elsewhere. It requires real focus and energy to stay aware and available to the person in the interaction, without thinking about plans for the rest of the day or some niggling worry over something said yesterday.

I came to mindfulness practice after downloading a meditation app, simply to get me through the jet lag from flying out to visit family in the States. Then the habit stuck and I started to notice the value. I started to realise that it might have a benefit to my work, too. I made small shifts in how I would prepare for therapy sessions. Instead of scanning through plans one more time, I started spending my last couple minutes before a session sitting quietly and noticing my in breath and out breath. Now, this practice has transferred to my SaLT preparation.

Once the toys are tidied away after each session, I remind myself of the next child's notes and then set a timer on my phone and lean back in the soft chair. (When you work with kids, you'll know how most of your working time is spent on the floor, so sitting in a 'proper chair' feels like a luxury worth taking.) For those couple of free minutes, I take a deep breath in and then exhale deeply, feel my feet on the ground, notice my belly moving with my breath, listen to the sounds around. This moment of mindfulness helps me feel a little more centred and alert when I greet the next family into the space.

There are many different prompts and models out there to help you try out some mindful breathing practice. Box breathing is a nice simple one to try. (Figure 6.1).

When we find moments to pause and notice our body in space, it helps us share that space with others all the better. It seems to me that children with little spoken language are very embodied: less lost in thoughts, more actively in their bodies. A big part of how they interact with the world is through movement: interpreting and coding what they see in others, exploring how they can move their own body in space. So it's useful to take a moment to become more embodied myself, less tangled in my endless thoughts or plans, more able to meet the child in the mode that they're already in.

CHOOSE YOUR FOCUS

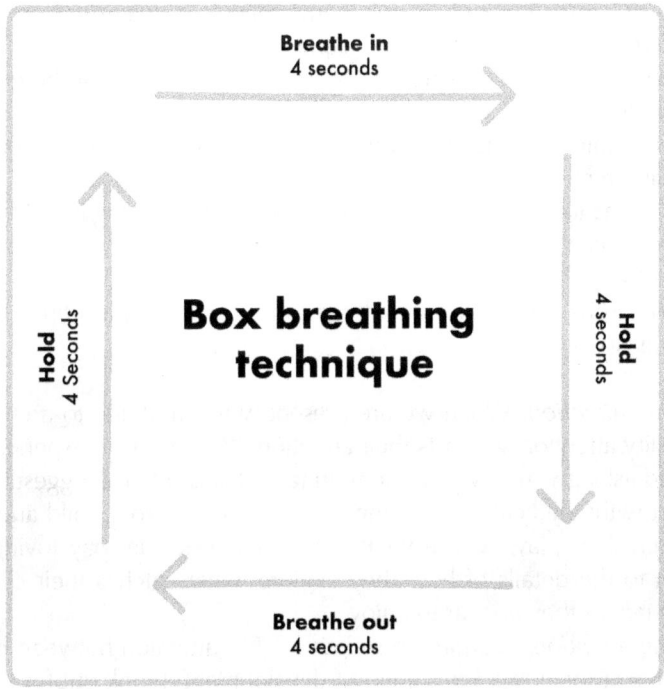

Figure 6.1 Box breathing technique

Mindfulness has benefits for our wellbeing, our ability to sustain our work long-term, to be able to genuinely show up for people in the way that we would like, as our full selves.

There are also benefits for our kids. When we look at some of the definitions of mindfulness, we can start to see how closely aligned they are with many of the interaction strategies that the research tells us benefits communication development.

Bishop et al. (2006) define mindfulness as: 'Self-regulation of attention (skills of sustained attention, switching, inhibition of secondary elaborative processing) and orientation to experience (curiosity, experiential openness, and acceptance).'

When I relate this to my own practice in supporting children through playful interactions I spot the similarities:

- paying close attention to what the child is doing, switching readily between activities as the child explores
- avoiding second guessing and overthinking so that I can be genuinely child-led
- approaching the interaction with an open curiosity and acceptance of what the child is doing
- not trying to change the play or direct it, but embracing it and following where I can

Let's look at the details of mindfulness as it relates to supporting children's communication:

Sustaining attention. When we are present, we can attune to a child. Our quality attention supports their attention. It's the classic experience of a child asking you to watch them. In fact, this is often a suggestion that I start with: Dedicate some time to sit down with your child and simply watch their play. Notice what they're interested in, pay loving attention to the details of how they explore, what catches their eye, what sequences they appear to enjoy.

Switching attention. Learning to switch or shift attention between different points of focus is a key aspect of development. I look out for it in children: how they shift attention, what causes them to switch. As adults, we also need to practise the switch. If we agree, as we discussed in Chapter 5, that following the child's lead is helpful, then we need to be able to switch our attention readily. We need to be able to abandon our ideas of what should happen next, to move and shift to whatever the child plays with.

Inhibiting secondary elaborative processing. This is simply another way of saying: 'Don't overthink it.' The moment we start elaborating and extrapolating on what the child is doing in the moment (what that might mean, what we should do next, whether what we're doing is any good) then we've entirely lost it. We're no longer attending to the moment. Instead, we're in our heads, busy thinking about it.

Orientation to experience. I aim to approach my sessions with curiosity, openness, and acceptance, so I was interested to see these three words used by Bishop et al. (2006) to describe aspects of mindfulness. Certainly, acceptance can be the hardest one in life and in practice.

I want our kids to experience wholehearted unconditional acceptance for how they are.

I've heard it said: 'If you don't have time to meditate for five minutes, then you need to meditate for ten.' The suggestion being that you need a meditation practice all the more if you live a life that gives you a sense of rushing and a lack of time.

I'm imagining you there, reading this page, burdened with your enormous workload, endlessly busy family life, and I hear you saying: 'Of course I'd benefit from a little quiet time to settle and regulate and turn up fully energised and attentive for our time with our kids. But amidst the emails, the schedules and the errands, when do I have the time for that?' We're tied into existing structures and lifestyles that demand this busyness from us so much of the time.

I mentioned this challenge to a parent recently, who I saw again years after working with her and her son. I expressed my shame-facedness at suggesting to parents they spend some quiet attentive time with their kids, when I can only imagine how busy their lives are.

She gave me a response that I wasn't expecting: 'The focused time that we did find together was only possible because you joined us.' Her comment created a shift for me, away from my fear of setting parents expectations that they couldn't possibly meet, and towards being an ally in helping them create pockets of possibility for slowing down, tuning in, and building interactions together.

This mum went on to say that the habits established through that early practice continue to influence her relationship with her now-teenage son. This felt like a celebration for me of the work that we do in the early years, its potential for long-term impact. I was struck by how this mum focused on the relationship built, the habits of quiet listening and attentiveness. She didn't start with 'He now has an excellent vocabulary', or 'He's on the debate team'. She valued the culture in their relationship that had been established by these early habits, learning to value and prioritise what's possible when we allow space to think and share. Decide what's important.

Creating a sense of quality attention and space to think is the majority of the work. Like so many things, the simple part is also the hardest part. That said, it is still only part. So let's look at some details: what we pay attention to, what we're looking for, and how we might respond in a helpful way.

Understand where the child's at

In speech therapy training, we're taught how to assess a child, so that we can report on their current levels, measure how far behind the 'norm' they are, and know what we need to focus on to help them out.

From a communication perspective, we specifically want to know about:

Attention. Can they maintain attention, can they shift attention, can they pay attention to others?
Understanding. Can they point to things when asked, can they follow spoken instructions?
Talking. Can they name things, can they name actions, can they construct sentences?
Speech sounds. Do their words sound clear, can they pronounce all the various speech sounds in our language?

Building this profile helps us to understand the aspects of communication that need some support. Do we need to help a child explore more varied speech sounds or some useful words? Perhaps we notice that sharing attention is tricky, or following routine instructions is hard. It's useful to have a focus for what we choose to model or pay attention to. We want to know what 'success' might look like for the child, so it's understandable to want to set goals. Truth is, I have a mixed relationship with goals. I see their benefit but I also experience their limitations.

Goals are useful for a number of reasons. They help us to:

- know what to focus on
- plan our time together
- show others we're proactive in helping a child
- measure progress over time
- monitor and adjust plans as we go
- enable teamwork – coordinate our efforts
- prepare a child for a point of transition, e.g., starting school

In my speech therapy training, we were taught to set SMART targets for each child to achieve:

Specific. Includes details of what you expect the child to do.
Measurable. Gives us a definite number or a clear yes/no answer.
Achievable. Can be achieved within the timeframe set.
Relevant. Is meaningful and useful for the child's long-term progress.
Time-bound. Has a clear timeframe in which the target is to be achieved.

I followed the protocol of assessing the child, identifying the problem, and then setting out the very specific new behaviour I expected to see in the child after a period of work.

That protocol would look something like this:

1. Identify what the child is not doing or *should* be doing in line with typical expectations for their age. e.g., *Child is only using nouns and not using verbs.*
2. Identify what a next step could be. e.g., *Child should be using verbs in order to construct full sentences.*
3. Break down that 'should' into manageable steps and create a target.

The goal might look something like: "By the end of the month, Anthony will use at least three verbs correctly within structured 1:1 activities with a supporting adult."

You could look at the goal-setting process another way:

1. Get to know the child, understand their strengths and needs.
2. Talk with the adults around the child, what they notice, what questions they have.
3. Agree together the focus areas for support.
4. Shape these into actions we can take to promote success.

I've become increasingly ambivalent about prescribing specific targets for a child, for two reasons:

1. When we're focused on a specific step, we can miss/undervalue/be unresponsive to the unexpected things that arise. That's a great loss, because what can't be measured is hugely valuable. Things like wellbeing, motivation, engagement …
2. Goals that are focused on the child's behaviour prioritise the wrong thing. Improving how the adults around a child are responding and interacting with the child can have the biggest impact, so we need to set goals that prioritise this. In others words, we need to create goals for the adults.

Write goals for the adults, not the child

The relationship between the child and communication partner is a crucial element of any communication goal, given that communication always requires at least two people (even here, dear reader, this writing is nothing without your reading).

I was taught that targets should always be about what we expect to see in the child. This was considered 'child-centred'. So I would diligently write targets that were about the specific behaviours I expected the child to demonstrate within a given timeframe. These goals put me in the position of prompting, directing, judging, coaxing to get the child to *do the thing*. Part of this came from the panic I'd imposed on myself about doing a 'good job', being worthy of my role.

If we acknowledge that children with communication difficulties need time and patience, then do our SMART targets really facilitate this? Or is it more pressure on the child to do more, a subtle persistent message that what they're doing already isn't enough? We've grown up with this message too, the fear that perhaps we're not doing enough. I suspect that's why I'm so often asked: 'How do I know when to push my child?' As the adult, whatever our role, we feel the expectation to push and drive the pace of progress, be doing *more*.

What would happen if we create goals that allow us to be in the interaction, joyful in the presence of the child, supportive of their growth, *without* judgement? I get that we want to be child-centred. All of us are in this because we care about the children we spend time with and have them at the centre of our focus for what we do.

But being child-centred can't mean that our focus is solely on what the child is doing. Communication isn't a solo act. We're a part of it. The way we respond and react shapes the moment. We need goals that encapsulate this dynamic, particularly if a large part of our focus in the early years is to facilitate learning through play, following the child's lead.

How does this fit into the statutory framework, the Early Years Foundation Stage (EYFS)? When you focus on goals that are about facilitating quality time, you are in a better position to provide the well-informed observations that the EYFS requires.

This means we want to create goals that help us be observant, rather than directive. Sometimes child-centred targets can look very directive. For example: *'Fatima will produce at least three different speech sounds when engaging in an activity with an adult.'*

I struggle with this wording. Who am I to dictate? It sets an uncomfortable tone and power dynamic from the beginning, this suggestion that I should know what's best. Friend and fellow Speech and Language Therapist, Kristy Ney, once suggested an idea that has spun in my head ever since: 'What if we view the child as the manual?' What if we believe that following and attending to the child gives us what we need to understand and support them further?

Here's an alternative way to frame that goal for Fatima: *Fatima is starting to show an interest in how she can make different sounds with her mouth. This is positive because it's an early building block for communication. We can help Fatima to develop this interest by noticing her speech sound attempts and acknowledging and/or copying these sounds.*

Many non-speaking children in the early years have tenuous communication skills, used rarely or only in specific contexts. A specific goal can highlight what a child is able to do 'sometimes' or 'almost' and make people alert to encouraging and responding to it. But, by setting a specific goal, there's a risk that we lose sight of the other things happening in the interaction. How can we truly notice the rich gestures and vocal pitch they're using if we're focused solely on whether they're saying 'Gruffalo' correctly?

One solution is to focus our goals on what we want to see in the adult rather than the child. We can have long-term goals for the child and get there through short-term steps and strategies for the adult (we'll get to a handy list of these in the next chapter).

When our goals capture an aspect of the adult's behaviour this helps us shift away from worrying about whether the child is 'getting it' and focus instead on the environment and learning what's helpful for the child.

Another element that can be really useful is to shift from writing SMART targets to ones that are a lot scruffier.

Write SCRUFFY goals

I came across SCRUFFY goals at a therapeutic storytelling workshop run by Louise Coigley, Speech and Language Therapist and founder of Lis'n Tell: live inclusive storytelling. I often grapple with goals (as you may have noticed from this chapter) and so I'm always keen to have conversations around the topic and hear alternative perspectives. Louise suggested that I investigate SCRUFFY goals, the work of Dr Penny Lacey.

Dr Lacey was a Speech and Language Therapist who worked with people with complex physical needs and learning difficulties. She was working within an education system that prescribed 'performance levels' for children who didn't meet the threshold for National Curriculum levels. Penny described how the SMART goals they were setting were very focused on small, isolated skills, repeated a specific number of times. Yet the problem was that the goals were not related to the student's point of interest and did not allow for flexible learning through exploration.

Instead, Dr Lacey drafted up an alternative acronym, only partly in jest:

Student-led
Creative
Relevant
Unspecified
Fun
For
Youngsters

She writes: 'SMART targets can be used effectively for learning the observable skills of counting e.g., rote counting 1–10. What is difficult for SMART targets to do is to support the learning of when counting takes place, why people count and what they can do with the counting once it is done.

SCRUFFY targets can be very helpful when building up understanding' (Lacey, 2010).

Let's take a look at another SMART target example: *'By the end of the month, Anthony will use at least three verbs correctly within structured 1:1 activities with a supporting adult.'*

This target is ultimately aiming for the child to have action words (verbs) as an option in his communication. The rest of the details in this SMART target primarily facilitates our record-keeping and confidence in marking a target 'achieved'.

If we were to make this target SCRUFFY it might look something like: *'This month, Anthony will have opportunities to explore actions when playing on the climbing frame, by doing and talking about it with a supporting adult.'*

It sounds so vague, it's almost uncomfortable. But think about how this would facilitate a focus between the adults interacting with Anthony: 'Action words, got it. Playing with stuff that he likes, looking out for the actions he makes, joining in with the actions, naming the actions.' We don't always need a more detailed map than this.

I'm interested in the benefit of being 'unspecified'. Being specific serves our need to *know* when we've reached the target. Being specific does not facilitate child-led learning. It doesn't allow for us to facilitate the spontaneous or unexpected moments of progress, the things along the way.

This is an idea that I first came across when working with Julie Calveley, a Registered Learning Disability Nurse, specialist in interaction and emotional wellbeing. She is also the founder of NAC, Nurturing Affective Care, a non-profit organisation dedicated to promoting the emotional wellbeing of children and adults with severe and profound disabilities. Together, we were exploring the ways that intensive interaction strategies were supporting a young girl's communication development.

Julie and I met regularly and, in every discussion, I would introduce the topic of goals. I wanted to be clear in my mind about what we were aiming for and make sure I was doing the 'right thing', making progress in a neat linear way. I was seeking the validation that comes with 'goals met'. I was also familiar with the importance of reporting on our progress against targets as part of communication with school. It made my work more comfortably correct if I had a neat summative table to share with school every half term. 'Look what we've achieved!'

Julie told me that, in intensive interaction, they don't set targets. Instead, they report on the progress they've observed. It got me thinking about how the very act of setting specific targets for children is a rather strange attempt at telling the future and potentially restricting what we notice and value. The act of setting a goal could even be seen as directive: We're expecting you to do this. It can shift us out of the present moment, when really the biggest practice for supporting emerging communication is to Be Here Now.

Julie explained to me how intensive interaction focuses on being attentive to, and curious about, the details of what we see an individual do in the moment. A little like being child-led.

If we avoid setting goals, or at least set only broad unspecified goals, we create the space to look out for the unexpected moments that spark curiosity in the child and inspire communication.

In many ways, SCRUFFY goals incorporate a greater level of trust for the child's intrinsic learning and ability to direct their attention towards their own growth and development. It focuses on opportunities to facilitate, gives the team a focus, perhaps informed by the child's point of interest or proximal development. This doesn't require the adult to be quantifying the child's progress and doesn't require prompting or focusing in on a specific detail.

Goals are important, but not nearly as important as the messy everyday playful interactions that we have with children. I'm far more interested in how you're spending time with the child, rather than how smart your targets look.

With that in mind, let's consider elements of a playful interaction that support connection and communication. These are relevant to all kids, but are all the more important for those at the early stages or those developing communication in a different way from the majority of their peers.

References

Bishop, S.R., Lau, M., Shapiro, S., Carlson, L., Anderson, N.D., Carmody, J., ... Devins, G. (2006) Mindfulness: a proposed operational definition. *Clinical Psychology: Science and Practice*, 11(3): 230–241.

Lacey, P. (2010) Smart and scruffy targets. *The SLD Experience*, 57(1) (June): 16–21.

7 A strategies list

In this chapter, we'll look at specific strategies that we can use within our interactions to support communication and connection. When trying out new strategies, it's useful to establish regular bits of 'practice time' throughout the week, perhaps five minutes a day. Creating some intentional, ring-fenced time is helpful when practising new skills. It's much harder to practice, and reflect on new strategies if you expect yourself to simply start doing it all the time. Once you establish some useful habits in these short moments of 'practice time', they can start edging in to the rest of the day. This chapter contains ten key strategies that are useful for establishing shared connection and developing communication with your child.

Figure 7.1 A list of strategies summarised in this chapter

DOI: 10.4324/9781003301967-7

Allow yourself to do less

When we're spending time with any child, it can be hard to adjust our pace to them. It can feel slow or non-productive. So, actively acknowledging the 'not much-ness' of it is important. This is an ongoing practice; be ok with it feeling quiet or slow. This is all the more important if you're feeling the urgency for your child to 'catch up' and 'start doing something'.

> TRY IT OUT: Can you spend time with the child where you prioritise tuning in to what they're doing, rather than trying to get them to do more? How does this feel for you? What do you notice? Chat through this with someone you trust. The insight it brings is an important part of helping us adjust to the individual child in front of us, especially if they aren't speaking.

Embrace the awkward silence

Sometimes, silence can feel like failure or not enough, perhaps disappointment, as we wish the child in front of us would simply start chatting away like we see their peers doing. If we can get over the initial discomfort of those long awkward pauses in conversation with a child, we create space for the child to lead.

As a supportive adult, learning to say less takes time. Keena Cummins, Speech and Language Therapist and creator of the VERVE child interaction approach, encourages us to imagine the finite airtime in an interaction. When we take up all the airtime with words and comments, there's no space for the child to say something. There's no need for them to fill the airtime because we're doing it for them.

The moments of silence while we give a child time to contribute can feel awkward because we aren't used to them. We're so used to chat, it can feel like there's something missing. But for kids, there's nothing awkward about it. In fact, it can be quite freeing to have a little more quiet, more time to think, more time to focus and form ideas.

When we break it down and consider each element of successful communication, as we did in Chapter 2, we can start to imagine how each step might take a child time, how they might benefit from a quiet attentiveness from us, rather than having us fill in every gap.

Embracing the awkward silence is one of my favourite strategies to use in all kinds of interactions through daily life. Silence feels awkward, for sure. But it's also powerful. If you embrace the moments of silence in any conversation, you will often find that people say more. They say things that are deeper and closer to the truth of the matter. With kids, these 'awkward' moments are actually busy with thinking. You're giving a child time to process, to consider what's happening, what they might like to do or say next. This then puts you in a great position to respond, rather than direct.

> TRY IT OUT: When silence crops up in a conversation, try counting how many seconds before someone speaks up. It's interesting to notice our tolerance for silence. If we can stretch this, we create more space for children to take the lead and make more attempts in their communication.

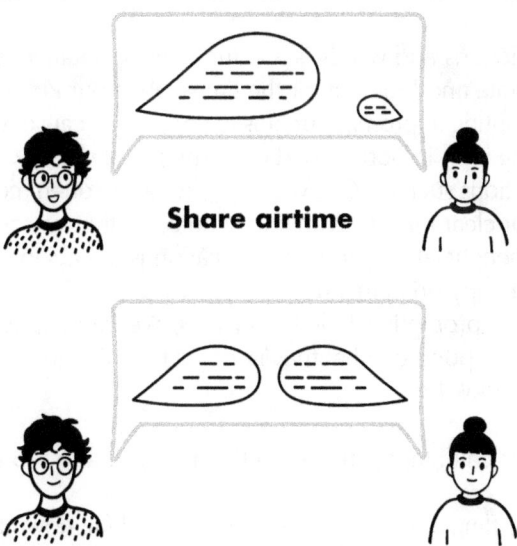

Figure 7.2 Balancing how much airtime we fill with words and sentences.

Reflect the child

In all our interactions, mirror neurones impact our behaviour. Without being aware of it, we will often mirror the expressions, actions, and gestures of our conversation partner.

This ability to notice another and reflect their actions is a part of the early interactions we have with babies. We accept all their sounds with delight and spontaneous imitation. We create balanced conversational turns with babies by responding to their babbling with the same sounds reflected back, or with brief utterances like 'Is that right?', 'Oh, wow!' etc. This helps babies explore and practise a valuable part of interaction and communication: reciprocity, as we each take a turn to bat our ideas back and forth to one another.

As kids get older and our expectations of them grow, it can be harder to maintain these balanced turns, particularly if the child isn't talking. We start to prompt or talk more or try to get something out of them. The simple act of acknowledging what they're doing and playfully reflecting it back to them can feel insufficient, as we wonder whether we should be 'teaching' more. There can often be the sense that we should be more directive if a child is going to learn.

Copying actions and words is a natural and spontaneous part of learning. We celebrate and look out for the times when our kids copy a word or phrase. It's tempting to prompt our kids to copy us, because we have a sense of how copying is an important part of learning. But when we approach our kids with questions such as 'Can you say___?', we're often met with an awkward silence or clear refusal. Even if they do copy, the very act of prompting makes it less beneficial. Key to communication is the ability to *initiate independently*, not copy on demand.

Rather than prompting kids to copy us, we can support our kids by copying them: respond to what they're doing by doing the same.

This might look like:

- when your child taps a finger on the mat, you also tap a finger on the mat
- when they fling a soft toy in the air to watch it fall down again, you also find a soft toy to fling in the air

A STRATEGIES LIST

We notice and acknowledge their actions by reflecting them back. We can do this with sounds, too. When a child tries a sound, or sings a tune, or attempts a phrase, we can reflect that back to them.

When we copy the actions, gestures, or sounds that a child makes, we are teaching them that their actions have an impact on the world around them, that they have agency and influence. This is crucial for non-speaking children, who can end up in more passive situations due to their lack of ability to talk about their world.

While copying is often the action described for this strategy, I prefer to think of it as reflecting. Reflecting is something we do in conversations and interactions with everyone, reflecting back their ideas, the key points of what they say, building on their contribution. To me, reflection suggests something a little more thoughtful. We don't want to just copy exactly what we see. Instead, we want to notice the details of what a child does and reflect that back in a way that feels like a response. It's about contributing to a back-and-forth exchange that feels meaningful and attentive. We're aiming to find a tone of unhurried acceptance and readiness to respond, which comes when we feel happily curious about what may arise.

This regularly involves letting go of our clear view on the purpose of a toy and instead reflecting what the child is doing with it. For me this week, that involved putting Woody into a zip-up bag and then opening the bag and tipping him out. The bag was actually storing a puzzle I'd brought to the home visit, but the zip bag, not the puzzle, was the thing that the child was interested in. He showed me that putting his Woody toy in the bag was interesting for him. I responded with phrases like: 'Zip it up!', and 'Hey Woody!' In my notes afterwards, I was able to report on his engagement and shared attention for the activity, plus some new sounds and phrases I heard him use. But, ultimately (and I believe most importantly), we had a whale of a time together.

> TRY IT OUT: Notice the moments when you want to direct the play in a certain direction, by pointing something out, shifting to something new, asking a question. Resist the urge! Instead, focus on what the child is already doing and try to reflect that back to them.

Pay attention to the details

When children are at the beginning of figuring out how to communicate with you, then small actions can mean big things. We want to pay attention to the details of what a child is doing, with their body, their face, their gaze, and more. All these details give us important clues about their thinking and their intentions.

What are they focusing on? What are they exploring? What specifically has caught their interest? Not just 'They're interested in the cars', not even 'They're lining up the cars', but all the little details: How have they chosen to arrange the cars? What parts of each car do they appear interested in?

Viewing with an imaginative lens, how might the child be experiencing this? Can you share in the appreciation of it? Tuning in to their point of interest and their perspective on the play equips us for how we respond. We can choose words and phrases that are really relevant and useful to the child, rather than shifting them out of their interest towards what we imagine they should or could play with instead.

Gather some short video clips of your play together, so you can pay attention to all the details and celebrate the moments of connection. Look at them closely; what's happening in them? I'm interested in spotting the moments of intention, when the child appears to have an idea, a desire, or an opinion. I'm interested in the moments when the child is successfully reaching out and telling me something.

If they are communicating a message, how are they doing it? Is it with sounds or gestures, or facial expressions? Perhaps, without words, they're saying 'I like this', or 'I don't like that'. Maybe they're saying 'Do it like this', or 'This thing is such fun!'.

Even if a child's message is 'No, don't do that', it's still important information. Sometimes, there's a negative view of these moments when a child says 'no' to us, but really it's such an important lesson for kids to learn. 'No' is a powerful word. It has impact and it can be a good starting point for a child learning that: 'My words make a difference.'

That moment of communication, or invitation to respond could look like the child doing the following:

A STRATEGIES LIST

- getting up close to my face and touching my lips, suggesting 'I'm interested in you/your face'
- vocalising distress because I didn't understand the child's plan and have done something they don't want
- handing me something
- doing something and then glancing back to see what I do in response
- forming a sound
- facial expressions
- looking towards us

> TRY IT OUT: Take a brief clip of you and your child (less than five minutes). Watch it back and jot down the details of what you see. Gestures and body positioning can convey a lot of information and give us clues about what a child may be feeling or thinking.

Play with words

Reflecting back what the child does is a valuable part of establishing and supporting early communication, but it doesn't end there. We also need to build and expand on it, to give them an increasingly rich variety of examples of things they can try out for themselves.

Having a core set of words and phrases in your mind can be helpful if you find your mind goes blank during play. This can happen if the play feels unfamiliar to you, or if you've been doing it for a long time and you've run out of things to say.

Back in my early days of running parent workshops in the NHS, we'd give parents sets of toys and ask them to jot down some things they might say about the play. Parents were often surprised by how hard this was, and it helped us all give ourselves a little more credit for the challenge of modelling fun words and phrases in the midst of play. It's worth experimenting with this kind of forward planning, to see if it creates more ease in play with your child.

As a simple starting point, think about what words would be interesting to your child. As vocabulary develops we can add more variety, not only

HOW TO HELP NON-SPEAKING CHILDREN IN THE EARLY YEARS

Word variety

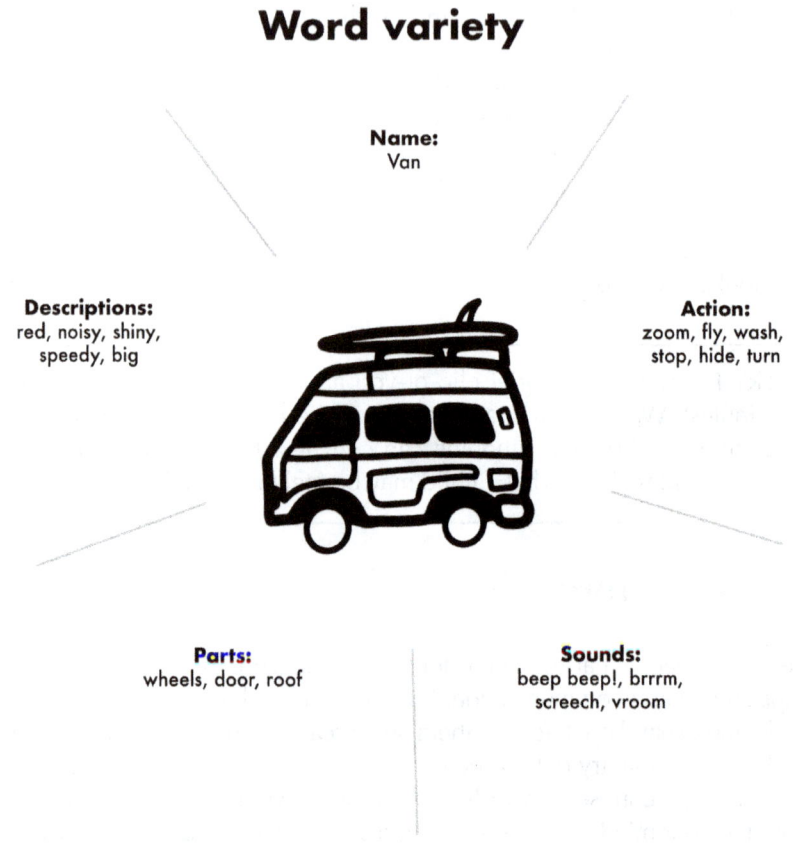

Name:
Van

Descriptions:
red, noisy, shiny, speedy, big

Action:
zoom, fly, wash, stop, hide, turn

Parts:
wheels, door, roof

Sounds:
beep beep!, brrrm, screech, vroom

Figure 7.3 A selection of some of the different word categories you might consider when adding word variety to your models

naming things, but also describing things, naming the specific parts of something, or giving some action words.

Jotting words down in this way can also help adults to be consistent, so the child hears some familiar phrases across different people and different situations. If you're making a list of some focus words, you could also add some phrases or sound effects, mentioned later in this chapter.

Think about the words or phrases the child might be using too. When a child is copying a phrase from a film, for instance, Buzz Lightyear's '100%

hyperspeed' that may be the child communicating: 'Let's throw things up in the air!', or 'Let's run really fast'. These phrases, learned and copied from favourite films or TV shows can sometimes be dismissed as meaningless repetition, the child 'stuck in a loop'. But that is a lack of imagination on our part, a lack of appreciation of the many and varied ways we can get our message across when we think laterally.

There's now much more talk about 'gestalt language processing', informed initially by the research of linguist Ann Peters and later taken up by Speech Language Pathologist, Barry Prizant. The key takeaway from their work is that not all children learn language by starting with individual words and then piecing them together to make phrases. Some children learn language as whole phrases, which they then break down over time to use the individual words flexibly and interchangeably to create novel sentences. You might not know if your child learns language as whole phrases or individual words, but that's ok! You can experiment by including some simple phrases in your play.

Think about what sounds, words, and phrases sound interesting. Think about the simplest phrase to convey the idea. If a child is really interested in how the cars go down the ramp of the toy garage, we could say 'vvvvroom!', 'weeee', and 'down'. We could also say 'Look at the cars!', or 'Down they go!'.

Once we have an idea of the words we could model, we also need to choose our moment carefully. Ideally, we're aiming to model a word or phrase at a moment when the child can take it on board. That comes down to timing and motivation.

Friend and fellow Speech and Language Therapist, Suzanne Churcher, often describes a child's internal word log (mental lexicon) as a filing cabinet, a concept she credits to her first mentor, Susie Brannon. When we model words that the child is interested in, at a moment when they're attending to us, it's like slipping the word into an open drawer, neatly filed for future use. If we're chatting away all the time, it's like throwing words at a closed stack of a drawers.

Picking our moments increase the impact of what we model. This is why we spend a lot of time prioritising shared engagement and responsiveness to what the child is telling us. That lays a good foundation for our being able to give useful words when the child is engaged in what we have to offer.

> TRY IT OUT: Consider an activity that your child enjoys. Jot down some words and phrases. Can you come up with something for every branch of the spidergram?

Use big gestures

Louise Coigley, Speech and Language Therapist, uses her skills as a dynamic storyteller to therapeutically engage and support the communication development of children and adults with communication challenges. When I attended Part 2 of Lis'n Tell: live inclusive storytelling training, Louise gave each of us a single word to gesture as we said the word out loud. *Rainbow, key, teapot, butterfly, banana* … As the participants each said their word, not only did they paint something beautiful and intentional with their hands, but the gesture itself seemed to enhance the way they said the word. Richer intonation, more emphasis and rhythm to the word.

Gesture is one of those no-brainers that we all have in our minds. We know that it's a key part of how we all communicate. Just try sitting on your hands while you talk. It changes things. Gesture is an important part of conversation, learning words and sharing ideas. Beyond even that, Louise's exercise made me realise what a really intentional and beautiful component of communication it can be. Since then I've paid far more attention and given greater celebration to the ways that children spontaneously or intentionally use gestures to communicate their ideas, with or without spoken words attached. I've realised how my own intentional use of gestures can support a child's attention, understanding, and opportunity to copy and learn from me.

Just last night, my husband asked me to explain the word 'attenuate' and then commented on how my explanation was filled with this particular pulling or 'stretching out' gesture that I was making with my hands. So, even for myself and my own learning, gesture is hard-coded into my vocabulary development.

If you're thinking 'Got it, Bryony – I'm all over it because I already use Makaton and everyday gestures', that's great *and* please consider this idea more, because it's not just about simple signing and pointing. My invitation today is to think bigger and broader. Don't just use gestures in your interactions with children; use *big* gestures.

> TRY IT OUT: Pick some of the words from your spidergram. Then, try out a gesture as you say each word. Think about making the movement from your shoulder, not your wrist. Paint the air with your sweeping gestures. How can you use your whole body to support the gesture?
>
> Don't rush! It's important to say the word as you gesture. You may notice how the gesture changes the way you say the word or perhaps your facial expression; this is part of the magic of gestures.
>
> Try it with a friend or colleague. Share with each other what you notice. I hope you'll also end up having a good giggle; that's how we get those synapses firing.

Make your phrases sing

In working with non-speaking children over the years, I've learned to have increasing appreciation for the musicality of language. Some of the phrases we use with children have a natural sing-song flow to them. Say to a child something like 'Oh dear!', 'Ready, steady, go!', 'All gone', 'Where'd it go?', and you'll likely find its half-sung, rich in rhythm and intonation.

Gina Davies, Speech and Language Therapist and creator of the Attention Autism approach (which starts with an activity fondly known by many children as 'the bucket') takes the concept of songs further. She encourages us to create 'Signature Songs': to build on the natural attention that children have for songs and add in more language that is relevant to everyday activities.

A signature song is a song that you know really well, so it easily flows from your tongue, with lyrics adjusted for the activity. The one that always springs to my mind is 'Here We Go Round the Mulberry Bush', with its familiar refrain: 'This is the way we [insert action here].' A signature song doesn't have to be a nursery rhyme. If Daft Punk or Swiftie are the tunes that live rent-free in your head, then perhaps you could create a version that's relevant to the whirl of the washing machine, or pouring milk into your cereal bowl:

'Wash the, t-shirts
Wash the, towels
Harder, better
Washing machine'
(Sung to Daft Punk's 'Harder, Better, Faster, Stronger')

'Cause I gotta find a bowl, bowl, bowl, bowl, bowl
And I'm pouring in the oats, oats, oats, oats
Baby, I'm just gonna pour that milk right in so
Pour it in, pour it in!'
(Sung to Taylor Swift's 'Shake it Off')

When we create little ditties about our everyday routines with kids we're doing two things:

1. crafting consistent repeated phrases, which help children learn language, particularly if their style of language learning is through whole phrases rather than individual words
2. creating catchy moments of language practice with a child, within everyday routines. The routine prompts the language-rich sing-songy moment. We create opportunities for a child to hear us say/sing something that they can listen to and maybe even join in

> TRY IT OUT: Pick a chorus or phrase from a song that you love singing. Then pick an everyday routine. Maybe it's emptying the washing machine, or buckling the car seat. Can you craft a song about that thing? Share it with others who do that thing with your child and you've created a consistent language routine within the everyday.

Use sound effects

Creating simple and appealing sounds with our mouths is a way that we can share early 'talk' in a way that is engaging for an early communicator. Gina Davies, mentioned above, often emphasises how important it is to be interesting, to be worth paying attention to. Adding more sound effects is a way to do this. It also gives children a way to understand and join in with the 'conversation' without relying on words.

We naturally create sound effects when we play with cars (vvbrrroom, beep!) or talk about animals (moo, meow!) But what about the washing machine (bedoof bedoof) or the kettle (blub blub)? Your child will give you clues about the sounds they're interested in. They might even give you some ideas for sound effects to match.

> TRY IT OUT: Notice the everyday things that your child is interested in. Get playful and try out some different sound effects to go with that. The more you play with this, the more you'll get a sense of what's interesting to your child. Bonus point if you can pair the sound with a gesture!

Give, don't quiz

You know those awkward conversations, the kind where you feel like you're not getting much from the other person? You keep throwing out chat topics in the form of questions: 'What's your week been like?,' 'Seen anything good on TV?,' ' Been anywhere fun recently?,' 'Looking forward to the summer?'

You find yourself searching around for question starters because the person you're with gives so little back.

It's understandable that we do this with our kids, too. If we don't get comfy with periods of quiet in play then we often fall into rapid fire questioning: 'What's that?' 'What are you doing?' 'What colour is it?' 'What are you looking at?'

We often use questions as an attempt to get more out of someone. I'm not sure if that's ever a successful strategy. (I know when I'm asked a lot of questions I say even less, especially if I'm not in the mood to talk.) It certainly isn't successful with kids who are still grasping a handful of first words.

Instead of quizzing for language give your child language: 'Oooh that's a big tractor', 'Wow, you're jumping!', 'It's blue!', 'You choose: apple or banana?'. All these examples include useful and specific language. Children learn the phrases they hear the most. I can't tell you how many kids I meet who are really good at saying 'What's that?' Sure, they might be curious and asking for someone to name something for them. But also, a lot of the time, it's simply the phrase they've heard modelled most consistently.

> TRY IT OUT: Look for things that you can give a child in your interaction. Things that are interesting to them that they might like to try out themselves. What are the main actions? Could you pick a big gesture to go with that? What are the interesting parts? Are there any hilarious or notable sounds during the activity? How could you imitate that sound yourself?

Make it easy

In Chapter 2, we talked about the reasons why 'laziness' isn't the reason for children not talking. It's easy for us to underestimate the complex challenges and effort involved in communication, particularly for a child whose brain is wired in a different way from the majority of the people they interact with. When we think 'Maybe they're just lazy', it's natural to think the answer is to then push them to 'Say the word' or not accept their communication attempts until they do it 'properly'. Here's an alternative: Make it easy!

When things feel doable, we're naturally more motivated to do them. Our kids who struggle to communicate are working outside their comfort zone way more often than their peers.

By making things easy for them, we're giving them more experience of success, which in turn encourages more communication attempts.

There are three main areas where we can make communication easier for children:

1. Easier to attend: turn off background noise, follow what they're naturally interested in, seize their moments of interest, be flexible to facilitate active engagement.
2. Easier to understand: use gestures, objects, pictures, movements, to back up your words and give visual clues about what you're saying.
3. Easier to express: accept everything (so the attempt becomes less scary), allow space, offer the word if needed, give don't quiz.

Eye contact: A word of caution

When chatting with parents and practitioners, eye contact is often raised as an important factor in a child's communication and social engagement. From a neurotypical perspective, this is understandable: eye contact in conversations can give us a sense of connection and shared understanding. But that's not the case for everyone and our experiences of how comfortable eye contact feels can vary a lot.

Expectations and norms around eye contact vary according to context. I'm regularly outed as a country bumpkin in London due to my habit of looking people in the eye and smiling. My brother, a long-time London resident, tells me it's not the done thing, but still I persist because it makes me happy. Eye contact, when to use it, how much is 'appropriate', is context dependent and really, just like personal space, quite unique to each individual in terms of what feels comfortable.

I've met many kids who can find it genuinely uncomfortable to sustain eye contact. One seven year old told me: 'It just feels wrong.' I want the kids I support to feel *right* in themselves. I don't want to teach them to do something uncomfortable when eye contact is something that varies across individuals and contexts. It's hugely important that our children learn that if things feel 'wrong' in their body, they can tell us and we will honour that.

The problem is, that if a child doesn't make eye contact, then they can sometimes miss moments of connection or not have their message heard and noticed by others. If eye contact is a valuable cue for us to respond to a child, then we need to consider how we adjust this for those children who don't use direct eye contact.

Consider the other ways a child seeks to connect with you in a conversation, or leaves space for you to add something. Look for why they gaze, for clues about the child's point of attention. The kids I've interacted with over the years have taught me that often kids are listening and engaging, even when I think they're fidgeting or looking elsewhere. Body language isn't always a reliable and consistent language for everyone, so we can't assume they aren't listening.

8 Keep going

Imagine something different

If you picked up this book, then you're probably in the middle of figuring out a child who is communicating differently from many of their peers. When you look at the children around you, perhaps you see a contrast in their development. Your child might be taking longer to learn things, or might be approaching things differently. This means that we have to imagine something different, too. If we focus only on the typical path that we imagined, then we see only the ways in which we're not on it.

The day that I left my big council job to set up independently as SaLT by the Sea, my husband and I drove to the dog shelter and met our dog, Rolo. I had such picturesque plans for our lives with a dog at home. I pictured this gentle companion who would sit quietly by my side at cafes and pubs, trot amiably along while I skated the seafront. I pictured sociable lunch breaks with other dog walkers, camping adventures, and trips on the ferry. Whatever the rose-tinted merry montage of having a dog might include, it all flashed through my imaginings as we drove home from the rescue centre on that first day with Rolo in the back seat.

Reader, it did *not* turn out like I imagined. Instead, I found myself grappling with a dog who was so afraid of the world, he lunged and barked at everything: plastic bags, buses, men in high viz jackets, other dogs, and dozens more unexpected things. Tom and I had to tag team our walks around the block, one of us scouting ahead for 'dangers' (i.e., almost everything). Needless to say, we didn't go to the cafe. We didn't have sociable lunch breaks in the park. He was not chill.

I found it so tricky. I cried a lot, told Tom how it was too hard, I couldn't do it. We watched all the YouTube videos on managing reactive dogs. We had dog trainers come and go, try everything from bribing with cheese to shouting down in gruff tones. They'd leave us with action plans that felt so doable when they were in the room and once they left us to it, every task felt suddenly impossible, unrepeatable. Even if it felt like we were getting somewhere for a minute, once I was alone with Rolo and trying to remember those training plans, I found myself facing him and feeling so lost, so useless.

That was many years ago. Nowadays, we do get to take him to the cafe and the pub. We do have our sociable lunch breaks and chats with people in the park. I even take him into the office with me and everyone marvels at what a good boy he is: 'So quiet', 'So chill'. I just smile and say: 'You have no idea.' He's made so much progress, we forget how hard it was back then. But it wasn't an overnight fix. It was hours and hours, week in, week out, of trying and failing. Tom and I would engage in these big debrief sessions after a walk gone wrong. It was easy to get stuck in cul-de-sacs of blame, judging our management of a situation, trying to navigate a way to learn from one another and talk it through, without leaving the other person feeling like shit.

We worked it out together, bit by bit, being kind to ourselves whenever it felt impossible. We started imagining a different story about what our lives with a dog looked like, where the moments of fun and appreciation came from. In the early days, I had to let go of my picture of a chill cafe dog, because that was not the dog I got. Rolo was something else entirely and I learned to appreciate what he was.

Thanks to him, I discovered every hidden gem of deserted forest and coast in my county. I learned the joy of being out for hours, learning to read another animal, and finding companionship in how he communicated with me. I loved watching his moments of bravery and trust. Tiny steps of progress became big moments to celebrate. We walked past a bus and he didn't bark! He sniffed a discarded plastic bag without freaking out! We found games he could play, places we could take him to, the people we could hang out with, the ones who were cool with him jumping up to say hi, or barking his bonce off at the postman mid-conversation.

The things Rolo can do now, the ways he can be in the world, might seem small to others, but we know how hard won they are. We've seen how much each step of progress improves his life and ours. We took him to a local artisan Christmas market at the end of last year, just casually walking around the stalls, and chatting with people, navigating like a smooth rider. Looks like no big deal to the people who don't know.

Rolo's road to get here looked so different from the puppies around us, and, in many ways, it still is. It's also bloody marvellous. He is a unique and tiptop excellent dog who brings us a whole heap of joy and appreciation for all the world has to offer.

When you're in the middle of something tricky, it can feel like it'll never change. When you're expecting things to go one way, but they head in a different direction, it can feel like a personal failing. Part of the journey is simply acknowledging that it's different than we imagined. And finding ways to write joy into this story.

What if we allow ourselves to imagine into the gaps of the conversations we have with non-speaking children? What if we allow ourselves a sense of rich conversation, true exchange and connection with this fantastic person? There are so many ways to have a conversation. You and your child are just getting started.

Let's start from a place of already enough. Turn up to each conversation without expectation, without a need for there to be more of something. It changes the quality of our attention, creates a better sense of connection. We humans long for belonging and this is something we're in a position of helping others find. A sense of acceptance, contribution to the group, ideas heard. It's small, and it's everything.

We're in the business of relationships

In speech therapy, we could say we're in the business of words, but really it's a matter of relationships. We want to spark meaningful connections with people that ever-so-slightly alters how they view themselves, the course of their contributions in the world. We're here to show them that their voice matters, however it comes out, that their ideas are important and interesting, worth taking the time to express.

In a culture stretched for time, if you have a sense of not enough, prioritise the relationship. Prioritise sitting with the child, the parent, and showing you care. Not about getting out a particular word, but about them as a unique and marvellous human. I hope we give families a sense of connection to their community, to each other and an affirmation of who they are together.

The simple version

If someone were to ask me in the street how we can truly help kids learn to talk, to speak their ideas to the world, I would tell them this: Wait, stop talking so much, pause for a moment! Can you settle into their pace, get a sense of what this child is thinking, and what they want to share with you? Can you notice how they share it?

Wait for your child to have the idea. Give them time to share it with you, with a point or a gesture, a look or a hunch, a 'huh', 'wow', or 'oooh'! Notice the moments a child invites you to join in and reply. Know and come to appreciate that it is about so much more than words. It's about how we respond with warmth, how we welcome more of those early moments of communication. We encourage by simply accepting all they give us, without correction or direction; 'Oh really!', 'Yes, I see that too.'

We're teaching children this: 'However you want to play, whatever you want to say, I'm here for it.' I could guess the ways that you may end up playing together, thinking back to times I've had: back and forth with a child, each making sounds like a fast game of ping pong. Throwing toys high up in the air, or hiding them under cups. Clapping, jiggling, laughing. Jumping into piles of cushions, dancing on coffee tables. (I'll leave you to do your own risk assessment.) Point is, you can't know where it will go.

Give them sounds and words and gestures like shiny tokens they can take and use themselves, or hold onto and stash away for a later date. I like to think of our kids with shiny collections of all the exciting and interesting sounds and songs that they've picked up from the adults around them.

I imagine kids saying to us (by a gesture, word or more): 'Now tell me about this, that looks interesting!' 'I love how this does the thing and especially when you look at it through this way or at this angle. Will you look at it with me?' 'Will you sit and watch while I sort these toys into ways that are uniquely joyous to me? Will you stay even if it looks like nothing?'

I'd ask them to give words, rather than quiz for answers. I'd tell them about what fun it can be when we aren't in charge, what unexpected moments of silliness and belly laughter come from just letting go of our plan.

And then I'd want to acknowledge what a powerful part of the progress comes from simply showing up. Sometimes, it feels joyful and we have a clear sense of progress. Other days, it can feel uncertain and stuck. It's all normal, it's all ok.

Share with others

All this stuff takes effort, cognitive and emotional. So, it's important to be able to talk it through: to make better sense of it, value the details, work through the moments of overwhelm. Find your community of folks who can talk these things through with you, help you grapple with the challenges and points of confusion.

Consider the experiences that prompted you to ask for help. Why now? Whether it's the family party that your child found overwhelming, or the frustrations of not being able to ask for things, thinking about the specific elements that make situations tricky can help clarify what would help.

When I get parents together for my Toddler Talk course, I allow a lot of time for sharing and listening to each other. I didn't initially plan for that, but I saw how often parents were keen to pipe up and say 'That's just like my kid!', 'My daughter does the same thing!'. I could see how they lit up from being part of a group that were experiencing similar things. Without these groups, families of non-speaking kids can feel always in the minority. Our support doesn't have to look like teaching or giving advice. As a Speech and Language Therapist, I'm often in a unique position to bring together families who might relate to one another. Do you know people you could bring together? Might you be a bit of a community match-maker?

Chatting with others helps you decide what progress looks like. It's in talking through your experiences and frustrations that you can clarify what kind of change you're hoping for. Consider the situations that feel tricky; what kind of change would help? This is where having a good listening partner is so helpful, because they draw out the details and save us from skating over things with broad generalisations: 'Ok, he gets frustrated ... give me an example. What does it look like?' Think back to the listening wheel. Are there questions on there that you could ask people to support them, or need to answer yourself? If things are hard, or even if they're not, make sure you talk about it!

Choose one thing

Just pick one thing from this book that sticks with you, and try that. From the ideas in the last chapter (and your own observations and hunches), pick an idea to focus on. Maybe you're going to ask fewer questions. Maybe you'll try some silly sounds, some gestures, or songs.

Maybe you're going to start a five-minute practice time, to sit down and focus on responding. What will you choose to notice and celebrate, encourage through the warmth of your response? Keep taking those video clips. Reflect on what you like about it, what you want to do more of. Scribble down those thoughts or questions. None of it has to look neat, or correct.

There are lots of ways that we can consider whether what we are doing is 'working'. We can observe and reflect, invite contributions from key people, track progress, keep records. And still, so much of what we achieve in relation to each other can't be known. So much of the value we gain from being with others can't be quantified.

I used to think that I was here to fix the kid. To get to the problem and solve it. But nowadays, I'm not convinced that anyone is broken. Communicating involves more than one person, so we can never place the problem within one individual. We share the challenge and we get better at it together.

The trick is having a sense of what's useful, and using specific strategies, building on what works between you and the child. But it's not just tips and ideas. There is a fair amount of heart with this, too. If you're going to keep going over a long period of time, you have to both enjoy spending time together and have a sense of the value in that.

Time spent together, building your connection and attention for each other is always time well spent. Be available, stay curious, allow things to be as they are. Allow play to go where the child takes it. What an experience this can give kids, this shift away from being prompted and told, towards a mode where they get to tell the tale, set the stage, lead their own story.

Stick with it

With an open and attentive mindset, and readiness to respond to what the child brings to the interaction, we can help our children to find their feet in the act of communicating. But that doesn't mean it'll be quick or easy.

We need to give time for things to take shape. We must keep showing up as a ready and attentive communication partner. We need to be there, to help them explore how we interact together, to figure out how to get a message across and how to receive the messages of others. At times, it's going to feel like slow progress. It's going to feel overwhelming and confusing. At other times, it's going to feel like things have clicked, like you can see where it's going. You'll notice more of the details in their communication and see these things happening more often.

Kids need us to keep showing up even when we feel like we're not doing a very good job. We can't control the pace of progress, or the many external factors that impact communication development. We can only control how much time we give something, what we pay attention to, how we respond.

The time that we spend with non-speaking children, attending to their things, viewing the world from their perspective, is time spent showing that child that they belong here, that their perspective and their contribution is valued.

The minutiae of the minutes you give to something is where your life is happening. All of this is in the tiny details. We think that change happens with big momentous decisions, great actions, and shifts in direction. But, really, it's about the everyday tiny choices that direct our course. One of my favourite reminders is from writer and activist adrienne maree brown: 'Small is all.'

Embrace everything

I didn't intend for surfing to become this valuable teacher for me. I just thought it was fun and wanted to keep doing it. But it's given me many parallels to draw on as I consider what it is for our kids to learn to communicate with us.

Words are like waves. Talking and surfing are both tricky skills to learn, but, on first glance, or from the perspective of someone who can already do it, they look easy. In surfing, the goal is to ride a wave. In speaking, we hope to hear words. And when your child is learning to talk, it's very easy to focus on the words. I've definitely been in SaLT sessions where I just want to hear that particular word a few more times. And I've definitely been out on my board, just wanting to catch one more wave.

Both words and waves can be so very few and far between. The number of waves that I actually manage to catch in a session might be pretty low. Like, two. Or sometimes none at all. If we made our reason for surfing to catch waves, or our reason to sit down with a child to hear their words, we could set ourselves up to feel pretty deflated. Because the count can be low. Instead, we need to find a way to appreciate and even enjoy every part of the picture. There's plenty happening below the surface. Without appreciation of the whole, we can end up a little lost.

It's often said that the best surfer out there is the one having the most fun. At times you're gonna look a fool and feel like you're making no progress, so half the skill is finding joy in the journey. That's how we keep turning up willingly, with wide-open grins.

If I only valued the wave-catching part of surfing, I probably wouldn't do it. The hours out there paddling, wiping out, or perched on a board looking at the horizon, are all far greater than the few seconds of waves caught. But I love looking up at the sky, how the light changes constantly, I love the different perspective it gives me on a familiar landscape. The soft feel of water tracing through my hands, the buoyancy of a wetsuit while I loll, watching others absolutely send it and whooping them on. I watch birds scoot past, notice the friendly faces around me, the cold water on my face. Knowing that I'm here for all that stuff too can help me to stay in it, even when it's tricky.

If you're helping a child communicate, be the ones having the most fun. Find the parts of it that make you grin. Tend to them, appreciate that here is where we find connection and figure things out together. We're learning to share in a child's world, spark joy together, delight in the details and advocate for what they need.

What are the parts that you can appreciate that make it ok to keep showing up even when it's hard? I love it when we end up giggling together. I love how often they explore a toy in a way I wouldn't expect. That 100-watt grin makes my day. The way that they move their hands, or bounce with excitement. The playful intonation in their voice or the side glance when they're thinking deeply. I'm paying attention to the moments when they make that sound, to the way they love the light pattern on the rug, or the way they join in when we sing that song.

Love what is. Love the half-formed word, the snail's pace. That's not accepting defeat, it's part of how we stay available, and make the next steps possible. Choose where to put your attention, because things blossom when we tend to them.

Truth is, it's entirely possible to feel lost when practising communication skills together. It often doesn't go according to plan. Our goals might give us the illusion of steady and predictable progress, but our lived reality often differs. Progress is messy and maybe that's ok. After all, we don't communicate always with the goal of making progress. That's not why we humans sit around and chat with one another.

A favourite childhood memory of time spent with my mum was this habit we had of sorting through coloured pens and playing with colour combinations. Teal and deep pink, sometimes paired with a pale grey. How much the pale pink and blue reminded us of spring, brown and yellow for a 70s' vibe. This satisfying loose parts play stuck with us as I grew up, from crayons as a kid to fineliner sets for high school exam revision. It facilitated conversations, this time that had no objective. It gave us just enough of a thing to do that we could sit there together and not get lost in our heads about what 'should' be happening. The moments that felt special were when we didn't have to achieve anything specific.

It's all in the noticing

In the month that I was finishing this book, we were just starting to emerge from winter. The days were becoming noticeably longer, not truly dark until gone six. Walking the dog around the steep bank of the local park, I passed the first of the pale green cow parsley, notable new greenness after our wet winter. As I noticed it, I got a strong whisper of its scent in my nose. I love whatever magical part of our noticing and interacting with the world around us makes our senses more alert to this stuff as we notice it. Yes, of course, the theory and particulars are important. And we might need to plan a structured use of visuals, coordinate support between services, analyse more data, but let's also remember how the world and people around us blossom under our attention. Just like the first green cow parsley's scent rose up to greet me as I noticed brushing past.

I think communicating can be one of the hardest things we ever do. It continues to be hard our whole lives. To say what we really mean. To say no. To stop saying sorry all the goddamn time.

I don't have any answers about communication. Just hours of seeing how children grow with attention and response, appreciation of who they are and who they become in an environment that loves their ideas, their attempts.

Developing the mindful qualities of attention, pace, and response, is a powerful foundation for our interactions. We can develop the tone of this over time, a practice where, just like mindfulness, the benefits are often intangible or filtered through the other things that you do.

Like the songs you sing together, the lyrics you make up.

The gestures you use to paint pictures in the sky.

The hilarious sounds or inside jokes that you share with your child.

The things that have you rolling around sharing a laugh together, or just sitting next to one another, quietly sharing space and knowing that there is so much in the times when it might look like you're doing nothing.

I wonder about how much we can perhaps know about one another and about ourselves when we take the time to sit down together, settle into a state of attentive presence, open to what might come, trying not to anticipate or direct it.

Commit to the everyday, see what comes. When you sit down with them, breathe and check in with yourself. You ok? Ok. What do you see? What are they doing? Don't judge. It's all ok. Your presence is a gift. Your warm acceptance of whatever they do, the responses you give, the gestures you carve. It's all good. Keep going. You're doing great.

Reference

brown, adrienne maree (2017) *Emergent Strategy*. Chico, CA: AK Press.

# Useful links

Gina Davies Autism Centre: https://www.ginadavies.co.uk/
Headspace app: https://www.headspace.com/
Intensive Interaction: https://www.intensiveinteraction.org/
Lis'n Tell: https://www.lisntell.co.uk/
NAC Wellbeing : https://www.nacwellbeing.org/
SaLT by the Sea: https://saltbythesea.com/
VERVE Child Interaction: http://www.keenacummins.co.uk

Acknowledgements

With huge thanks and appreciation to all the people mentioned in this book: colleagues, clients, and friends. And to those not mentioned in these pages, who read early drafts, gave valuable critiques and warm encouragement, and believed in my ability to write this when I didn't. I've learned so much from all of you.

Thanks to my editor, Clare, without whom I would never have attempted this project. And to the rest of the Routledge team who kicked into gear to make this happen and were always so responsive to my requests.

Thanks to my friend, colleague and illustrator, Victoria, who captured the heart of this project more than I could have hoped.

And to my husband Tom, always listening, always encouraging. I'm lucky to travel through life with you.

Finally, to Rolo, the rescue mutt, who snoozed patiently while I typed and only occasionally grumbled about needing dinner or a walk.

Thank you all and I love you!

Index

Page numbers in **bold** refer to figures.

acceptance 68–69
accepting interactions 33
actions: copying 80–81
active attention 3
active listening 27–30, **29**
advocacy: child needs 24
age-expected skills 39
agency: child 53
aims 1–2
airtime 78–79, **79**
appreciation 63, 100; culture of 45; moments of 35–36
assessment 47, 70–72
attention 102; active, 3; assessment 70; close 42, 82–83; giving 57–58, 66; quality 69; sustaining 68; switching 68
attention development 57
attentive presence 59, 102
awareness: expanding 10–11

babies 80
back-and-forth interactions 38
background noise 10, 91
beginnerhood: experience of 17–19
belonging: sense of 3

benefit of the doubt mindset 46–48
benefits 102
Bishop, S.R. 67, 68
blame 33
body language. see non-verbal communication
Box breathing 66, **67**
Brannon, Susie 85
breathing 31, 66, **67**
bridges 11
Burnham, J. 25–26, **25**

Calveley, Julie 75–76
capability 18
carers and caregivers: experience of acceptance and celebration 35–36; interaction skills 21; questions 24–25
celebration 39, 46; moments of 35–36
challenge: points of 26–27
change: potential for 41
child agency 53
child-led play 54–57, 60–61,
child needs: advocacy 24
child profile 70–72
children: inclusion 43; trusting 46–48
child's lead: following 13

105

INDEX

child's perspective 12, 17–19, 42, 54; tuning into 59
Churcher, Suzanne 85
clarity 44
close attention 42, 82–83
cognitive psychology 38
Coigley, Louise 74, 86
collaboration: relating through 27
comfort zones 51, 90
commentary 62
commitment: to the everyday 102
communication: child-centred 96; conceptualization 1, 6–12, **8**, **9**; difficulty 101; easy 15–16; fundamentals of 41–42; importance 1; interlinking skills 7–8, **8**; key 80; make it easy 90–91; mindfulness 11; misunderstanding 6; moment of 82–83; multimodal 9–10, **9**; opportunities 15–17; process 7; reasons for 14–15; riches of 15; shared 22
communication partners 21; inclusion 22–24
communication profile 40–42; focus on 44
communication skills: role 3
communication time 58
communicative attempts: sensitivity to 16
compassion 34–35
connection 2, 95, 100
consistency 23
contributions: valuing 26–27
conversation: building 64; experiences 6; initiating 15–16; quality 64; sounds 16; without expectation 95
copying 80–81
cultural reference points 23

Cummins, Keena 53, 78
curiosity 2

Davies, Gina 87, 89
details: close attention to 42, 82–83; noticing 12, 58
difference: frame of 44
difficulties: measuring 39
directing 54–55
disorder: language of 43–44
doing less 3, 78

early experiences 21
Early Years Foundation Stage 73
effort 97
emotions 59–60
empathy 2, 32, 34–35
encouragement 12
engagement 3; shared 10–11
enjoyment: shared 49
environment 18; physical **20**, 21; social 20, **20**
environmental processing demands 10
everyday routines: songs about 88
expectation: conversation without 95
experience 27; sharing 15
experience orientation 68–69
eye contact 53, 91–92

faces: interest in 62
family history 21
family support workers 45
favourite things: appreciating 47–48
fears 34–35
feelings 32
fix-it mode: avoidance of 30–32
flat hierarchy 24–28
focus 10–11
formal diagnosis 44

foundations 10
freedom: sense of 3
fun 17, 100
functional needs 15
fundamentals of communication 41–42

Gerber, Magda 63
gestalt language processing 85
gestures 86–87, 96
goals 10, 63, 101; child-centred 72, 73; framing 73; importance 76; long-term 73; SCRUFFY goals 74–76; setting 71–72; short-term 73; SMART targets 70, 72, 74–75; supportive 72–73; unspecified 75–76; usefulness 70; validation of 75

hands 10
harm: risk of 52
health visitors 35, 39
help: getting 97
Hewett, Dave 41
hierarchical thinking 24–28
honesty 24
hope: narrative of 37–40, **38**

ideas: building on 64–65; communicating 49–50; sharing 24
imaginative lens 82
inclusion 22–24, 43
input: valuing everyone's 22–24
inspiration: finding 6
intensive interaction 76
intention: moments of 82
intentional responses 3
interaction: flow of 12; foundation establishment 23; pace of 53; quality 64–65
interaction skills: caregivers 21

interest: sparking 10–11
internal reactions: noticing 6
invitations 53, 54

judgement 32–33

labels and labelling 43–44
Lacey, Penny 74
language 43–44, 45; conceptualization 7; giving 89–90; judgemental 45; modelling 56; musicality 87–88
language difficulties 7
language processing 85
laziness 90
learning 17, 55, 57, 80, 88
learning together 12
listening: active 27–30, **29**; to understand 30–32; value of 28
Listening Wheel **29**, 30
lived experience 28–29
long-term goals 73
love 33
love what is 100–101

make it easy strategy 90–91
mental lexicon 85
mindfulness 11, 65–69, **67**, 102
mindset 98
mirroring 80–81
mirror neurones 80
modelling 56–57
moment of communication 82–83
monitoring charts 39
motivation 15, 17
multimodal communication 9–10, **9**
musicality 87–88

narrative choice 37
narrative shifting 35, 37–40, **38**

needs: focus on 45–46
neurodiversity 44
neurology 21
Ney, Kristy 73
non-verbal communication 8–11, **8**, **9**, 12, 40, 92
notes 44
noticing 101–102

observations: sharing 27
openness 24
optimistic thinking 46–48
outsider experience 1–2
overthinking 68

pace: adjusting 78
parenthood: and judgement 33
parents: expectations 69; feelings 32; inclusion 22–24; struggle 33
patience 2, 53
pauses 58
performance levels 74
perseverance 98–99
perspective 27
Peters, Ann 85
physical environment **20**, 21
physiology 21
play: appreciating 47–48; child-led 54–57, 60–61, 96; directing 81; observing 49–52; plans 51; point of interest 61; as a teachable moment 55; types 61; understanding 22–23
play development 61
positive feedback loops 40
power dynamic 24–28
practice time: planning 16–17
predictions 31
priorities: deciding on 63–65
Prizant, Barry 85

process: joy in 37
processing demands: environmental 10
processing load 52–53
procrastination 65
professional relationship: building 32
progress 18, **19**; messy 101; pace of 99; potential for 37; tiny steps 94

quality attention 69
quality time: need for 35
questions 29–30, 89–90; carers 24–25; points of 26–27
quiet attentiveness 79
quizzing 89–90

reference points 22
reflecting 80–81
relationships 69, 95
repetition 23
resource access 21
resources: levels of 33
respect 44–45, 63
responding 12–13, **13**, 14, 50–51, 53, 54–57
responsibility 26
Rolo (dog) 93–95

scheduling 58, 59
SCRUFFY goals 74–76
primary elaborative processing: inhibiting 68
self-regulation 59–60
sensitivity 16
sensory information: processing demands 10
sensory profiles 10
shared attention 81
shared engagement 10–11
shared humanity 34–35

INDEX

shared moments 49–50
sharing 97
shortcuts 31
short-term goals 73
Signature Songs 87–88
silence 78–79, **79**; tolerance for 79
singing 22–23, 87–88
sitting alongside 50–52
SMART targets 71, 72, 74–75
social environment 20, **20**
Social GRACES framework 25–26, **25**
sound effects 22–23, 89
space: creating 52–53
special moments 101
speech: conceptualization 7
speech and language development: factors impacting 19–21, **20**
speech and language pathology 43
speech and language therapy: child led 2
speech difficulties 7
speech sounds: assessment 70
standard development 45
strategies 77, **77**, 97–98; attention to the details 82–83; doing less 78; gestures 86–87; give language 89–90; make it easy 90–91; practice time 77; reflecting 80–81; silence 78–79, **79**; singing 87–88; sound effects 89; word play 83–85, **84**
strength-based description 40–42
success criterion 17–18

support 97; levels of 33
supportive adults: role of 15

talking: assessment 70; challenge of 17–19; focus on 18
teachable moment: play as 55
terminology 43–44
therapeutic approaches: child led 2–3
thinking: optimistically 46–48
thinking time 52–53
time demands 58, 95
time giving 28
toy trap, the 61–62
tracking systems 39
trust 32, 76
tuning in 50–51
two-year check 35, 39

understanding 33; assessment 70; others 34–35
unexpected, the 72
unspecified goals 75–76
unspoken, the 33

video records 11, 42, 54, 82
vocabulary development 83–85, **84**

wellbeing 67
whole, the: appreciation of 99–101
word play 83–85, **84**
words: focus on 11–12

For Product Safety Concerns and Information please contact our EU representative GPSR@taylorandfrancis.com
Taylor & Francis Verlag GmbH, Kaufingerstraße 24, 80331 München, Germany

www.ingramcontent.com/pod-product-compliance
Lightning Source LLC
Chambersburg PA
CBHW050528170426
43201CB00013B/2128